Personalized Diagnosis and Therapy for Multiple Sclerosis

Personalized Diagnosis and Therapy for Multiple Sclerosis

Editor

Cristina M. Ramo-Tello

MDPI • Basel • Beijing • Wuhan • Barcelona • Belgrade • Manchester • Tokyo • Cluj • Tianjin

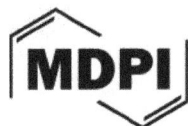

Editor
Cristina M. Ramo-Tello
Germans Trias i Pujol Hospital
Spain

Editorial Office
MDPI
St. Alban-Anlage 66
4052 Basel, Switzerland

This is a reprint of articles from the Special Issue published online in the open access journal *Journal of Personalized Medicine* (ISSN 2075-4426) (available at: https://www.mdpi.com/journal/jpm/special_issues/personalized_ms).

For citation purposes, cite each article independently as indicated on the article page online and as indicated below:

LastName, A.A.; LastName, B.B.; LastName, C.C. Article Title. *Journal Name* **Year**, *Volume Number*, Page Range.

ISBN 978-3-0365-5255-2 (Hbk)
ISBN 978-3-0365-5256-9 (PDF)

© 2022 by the authors. Articles in this book are Open Access and distributed under the Creative Commons Attribution (CC BY) license, which allows users to download, copy and build upon published articles, as long as the author and publisher are properly credited, which ensures maximum dissemination and a wider impact of our publications.

The book as a whole is distributed by MDPI under the terms and conditions of the Creative Commons license CC BY-NC-ND.

Contents

About the Editor vii

Preface to "Personalized Diagnosis and Therapy for Multiple Sclerosis" ix

Cristina Ramo-Tello
Personalized Diagnosis and Therapy for Multiple Sclerosis
Reprinted from: *J. Pers. Med.* **2022**, *12*, 1017, doi:10.3390/jpm12061017 1

Cristina Ramo-Tello, Yolanda Blanco, Luis Brieva, Bonaventura Casanova, Eva Martínez Cáceres, Daniel Ontaneda, Lluís Ramió-Torrentá and Àlex Rovira
Recommendations for the Diagnosis and Treatment of Multiple Sclerosis Relapses
Reprinted from: *J. Pers. Med.* **2022**, *12*, 6, doi:10.3390/jpm12010006 3

Bonaventura Casanova, Carlos Quintanilla-Bordás and Francisco Gascón
Escalation vs. Early Intense Therapy in Multiple Sclerosis
Reprinted from: *J. Pers. Med.* **2022**, *12*, 119, doi:10.3390/jpm12010119 15

Júlia Granell-Geli, Cristina Izquierdo-Gracia, Ares Sellés-Rius, Aina Teniente-Serra, Silvia Presas-Rodríguez, María José Mansilla, Luis Brieva, Javier Sotoca, María Alba Mañé-Martínez, Ester Moral, Irene Bragado, Susan Goelz, Eva Martínez-Cáceres and Cristina Ramo-Tello
Assessing Blood-Based Biomarkers to Define a Therapeutic Window for Natalizumab
Reprinted from: *J. Pers. Med.* **2021**, *11*, 1347, doi:10.3390/jpm11121347 29

Elisabet Lopez-Soley, Eloy Martinez-Heras, Magi Andorra, Aleix Solanes, Joaquim Radua, Carmen Montejo, Salut Alba-Arbalat, Nuria Sola-Valls, Irene Pulido-Valdeolivas, Maria Sepulveda, Lucia Romero-Pinel, Elvira Munteis, Jose E. Martínez-Rodríguez, Yolanda Blanco, Elena H. Martinez-Lapiscina, Pablo Villoslada, Albert Saiz, Elisabeth Solana and Sara Llufriu
Dynamics and Predictors of Cognitive Impairment along the Disease Course in Multiple Sclerosis
Reprinted from: *J. Pers. Med.* **2021**, *11*, 1107, doi:10.3390/jpm11111107 49

Elisabet Lopez-Soley, Jose E. Meca-Lallana, Sara Llufriu, Yolanda Blanco, Rocío Gómez-Ballesteros, Jorge Maurino, Francisco Pérez-Miralles, Lucía Forero, Carmen Calles, María L. Martinez-Gines, Inés Gonzalez-Suarez, Sabas Boyero, Lucía Romero-Pinel, Ángel P. Sempere, Virginia Meca-Lallana, Luis Querol, Lucienne Costa-Frossard, Maria Sepulveda and Elisabeth Solana
Cognitive Performance and Health-Related Quality of Life in Patients with Neuromyelitis Optica Spectrum Disorder
Reprinted from: *J. Pers. Med.* **2022**, *12*, 743, doi:10.3390/jpm12050743 61

Stijn Denissen, Oliver Y. Chén, Johan De Mey, Maarten De Vos, Jeroen Van Schependom, Diana Maria Sima and Guy Nagels
Towards Multimodal Machine Learning Prediction of Individual Cognitive Evolution in Multiple Sclerosis
Reprinted from: *J. Pers. Med.* **2021**, *11*, 1349, doi:10.3390/jpm11121349 73

Nupur Nag, Maggie Yu, George A. Jelinek, Steve Simpson-Yap, Sandra L. Neate and Hollie K. Schmidt
Associations between Lifestyle Behaviors and Quality of Life Differ Based on Multiple Sclerosis Phenotype
Reprinted from: *J. Pers. Med.* **2021**, *11*, 1218, doi:10.3390/jpm11111218 91

Nima Sadeghi, Piet Eelen, Guy Nagels, Corinne Cuvelier, Katinka Van Gils, Marie B. D'hooghe, Jeroen Van Schependom and Miguel D'haeseleer
Innovating Care in Multiple Sclerosis: Feasibility of Synchronous Internet-Based Teleconsultation for Longitudinal Clinical Monitoring
Reprinted from: *J. Pers. Med.* **2022**, *12*, 433, doi:10.3390/jpm12030433 . . . . **103**

About the Editor

Cristina M. Ramo-Tello

Cristina M. Ramo-Tello, MD (University of Zaragoza, Spain), trained as a specialist in neurology (12 de Octubre Hospital, Madrid), obtained her PhD on the treatment of multiple sclerosis relapse. She has dedicated her professional career to general neurology and multiple sclerosis. She is currently the Head of the Multiple Sclerosis Unit of Germans Trias i Pujol Hospital in Badalona, Spain. Her specialization and dedication to MS and neuroimmunology dates back to the 1990s. In terms of research topics, she has developed in particular the study of the treatment of multiple sclerosis relapse and the treatment of multiple sclerosis by the transplantation of autologous mesenchymal cells or by dendritic cells tolerant against myelin peptides. Her research lines are all funded by official national and European grants, which have led to doctoral degrees and international publications. Other lines of research include the search for diagnostic and prognostic biomarkers.

Preface to "Personalized Diagnosis and Therapy for Multiple Sclerosis"

This Special Issue reprint, entitled "Personalized Diagnosis and Therapy for Multiple Sclerosis", will help the clinician working regularly with people who suffer from multiple sclerosis (MS), thanks to the excellent work of all the authors who have contributed to its realization. This reprint issue offers key concepts, practical statements and a therapeutic algorithm seeking to standardize the care process for MS relapse, as well as a critical narrative review of the evidence to determine whether it is better to offer our patients escalation therapy or early intense therapy to prevent long-term outcomes. Biomarker research conducted by our colleagues evaluating CD49d saturation under natalizumab treatment can be used to optimize an individual's dosing schedule and thereby reduce the risk of progressive multifocal leukoencephalopathy.

From the clinical point of view, in this Special Issue we explain predictors of cognitive impairment, helpful to identify patients at risk, and also confirm the presence of cognitive impairment in patients with neuromyelitis optica spectrum disorder. On the other hand, we aim to boost the field of machine learning for cognitive prognosis that until now has been largely overlooked.

Because the patient is also the guardian of his or her own health, we must explain to the patient the evidence that lifestyle behaviors are associated with quality of life and encourage him or her to adhere to these behaviors.

Finally, the results of the studies carried out demonstrate that longitudinal clinical monitoring using real-time audiovisual teleconsultation over the internet is feasible and well-received by patients with MS and that such an approach can be a promising new care strategy not only in the short term but also in the long term.

We believe that the papers in this Special Issue reprint reflect our interest in conducting research for people with MS rather than conducting research about MS.

Cristina M. Ramo-Tello
Editor

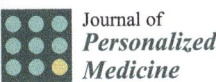

Editorial

Personalized Diagnosis and Therapy for Multiple Sclerosis

Cristina Ramo-Tello

Hospital Germans Trias i Pujol, Ctra Canyet, s/n, 08916 Badalona, Spain; cramot.germanstrias@gencat.cat

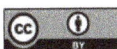

This Special Issue, entitled "Personalized Diagnosis and Therapy for Multiple Sclerosis" encompasses eight publications that we consider relevant, because their reading will help the clinician working regularly with people who suffer from multiple sclerosis (MS).

We all know that the primary interest of the neurologist treating a person with MS is minimizing his/her risk of having a MS relapse. Interestingly, the diagnosis and treatment varies greatly among clinicians and research in this field is very scarce. This issue offers a manuscript [1] with definitions of key concepts and a series of simple and practical statements with specific therapeutic recommendations, including an algorithm, seeking to standardize the care process for MS.

Currently there are up to 19 drugs approved to avoid the onset of relapses but there is no clear evidence to guide fundamental decisions such as what treatment should be chosen in the first place. This issue contributes a critical narrative review of the evidence on this still unresolved important issue, whether it is better to offer our patients Escalation Therapy or Early Intense Therapy [2] to prevent long-term outcomes.

One of the drawbacks of starting treatment with drugs of higher efficacy from the beginning is the less favorable side-effect profile. The search for biomarkers is essential to establish a personalized and safe medicine. Biomarker research conducted by some of our colleagues evaluating CD49d saturation under natalizumab treatment [3] has made it possible to make progress in this direction. CD49d saturation is a stable biomarker that can be used to optimize an individual's dosing schedule and establish a safety range to personalize the treatment and thereby reduce the risk of progressive multifocal leukoencephalopathy.

From the clinical point of view, the interest in the cognitive assessment of patients with MS has been increasing over the years. It has gone from being an undervalued symptom to one considered essential that requires continuous monitoring. In this Special Issue we are especially interested in cognition, and experts on the subject explain predictors of cognitive impairment helpful to identify patients at risk [4] and also confirm the presence of cognitive impairment in patients with neuromyelitis optica spectrum disorder and its impact on health-related quality of life [5]. On the other hand, it aims to boost the field of machine learning for cognitive prognosis because most investigations on machine learning for MS prognosis were geared towards predicting physical deterioration, while cognitive deterioration, although prevalent and burdensome, remained largely overlooked [6].

Physical and mental health is not only in the hands of the professionals, since the patient is also the guardian of their own health. As professionals we must strive to explain to the patient the evidence that lifestyle behaviors are associated with quality of life [7], advise them on those that best suit them, and encourage them to adhere to these behaviors.

Finally, we wish to thank the coronavirus crisis for the thrust it has given to the adoption of teleconsultation. The results of the studies carried out demonstrate that longitudinal clinical monitoring using real-time audiovisual teleconsultation over the Internet is feasible and well-received by patients with MS and that such an approach can be a promising new care strategy not only in the short term but also in the long term [8].

We believe that the papers in this special issue reflect our interest in researching for people with MS rather than researching about MS.

Funding: This research received no external funding.

Acknowledgments: We wish to thank all the authors who contributed their work, and in so doing made the Special Issue a success. We also wish to thank the staff of JPM for their excellent support throughout the editorial process.

Conflicts of Interest: The author declares no conflict of interest.

References

1. Ramo-Tello, C.; Blanco, Y.; Brieva, L.; Casanova, B.; Martínez-Cáceres, E.; Ontaneda, D.; Ramió-Torrentá, L.; Rovira, À. Recommendations for the Diagnosis and Treatment of Multiple Sclerosis Relapses. *J. Pers. Med.* **2021**, *12*, 6. [CrossRef] [PubMed]
2. Casanova, B.; Quintanilla-Bordás, C.; Gascón, F. Escalation vs. Early Intense Therapy in Multiple Sclerosis. *J. Pers. Med.* **2022**, *12*, 119. [CrossRef] [PubMed]
3. Granell-Geli, J.; Izquierdo-Gracia, C.; Sellés-Rius, A.; Teniente-Serra, A.; Presas-Rodríguez, S.; Mansilla, M.J.; Brieva, L.; Sotoca, J.; Mañé-Martínez, M.A.; Moral, E.; et al. Assessing Blood-Based Biomarkers to Define a Therapeutic Window for Natalizumab. *J. Pers. Med.* **2021**, *11*, 1347. [CrossRef] [PubMed]
4. Lopez-Soley, E.; Martinez-Heras, E.; Andorra, M.; Solanes, A.; Radua, J.; Montejo, C.; Alba-Arbalat, S.; Sola-Valls, N.; Pulido-Valdeolivas, I.; Sepulveda, M.; et al. Dynamics and Predictors of Cognitive Impairment along the Disease Course in Multiple Sclerosis. *J. Pers. Med.* **2021**, *11*, 1107. [CrossRef] [PubMed]
5. Lopez-Soley, E.; Meca-Lallana, J.E.; Llufriu, S.; Blanco, Y.; Gómez-Ballesteros, R.; Maurino, J.; Pérez-Miralles, F.; Forero, L.; Calles, C.; Martinez-Gines, M.L.; et al. Cognitive Performance and Health-Related Quality of Life in Patients with Neuromyelitis Optica Spectrum Disorder. *J. Pers. Med.* **2022**, *12*, 743. [CrossRef] [PubMed]
6. Denissen, S.; Chén, O.Y.; De Mey, J.; De Vos, M.; Van Schependom, J.; Sima, D.M.; Nagels, G. Towards Multimodal Machine Learning Prediction of Individual Cognitive Evolution in Multiple Sclerosis. *J. Pers. Med.* **2021**, *11*, 1349. [CrossRef] [PubMed]
7. Nag, N.; Yu, M.; Jelinek, G.A.; Simpson-Yap, S.; Neate, S.L.; Schmidt, H.K. Associations between Lifestyle Behaviors and Quality of Life Differ Based on Multiple Sclerosis Phenotype. *J. Pers. Med.* **2021**, *11*, 1218. [CrossRef] [PubMed]
8. Sadeghi, N.; Eelen, P.; Nagels, G.; Cuvelier, C.; Van Gils, K.; D'hooghe, M.B.; Van Schependom, J.; D'haeseleer, M. Innovating Care in Multiple Sclerosis: Feasibility of Synchronous Internet-Based Teleconsultation for Longitudinal Clinical Monitoring. *J. Pers. Med.* **2022**, *12*, 433. [CrossRef]

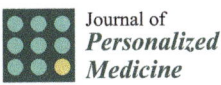

Article

Recommendations for the Diagnosis and Treatment of Multiple Sclerosis Relapses

Cristina Ramo-Tello [1,*], Yolanda Blanco [2], Luis Brieva [3], Bonaventura Casanova [4], Eva Martínez Cáceres [5], Daniel Ontaneda [6], Lluís Ramió-Torrentá [7,8] and Àlex Rovira [9]

1. Multiple Sclerosis and Clinical Neuroimmunology Unit, Germans Trias University Hospital, 08916 Badalona, Spain
2. Multiple Sclerosis Unit, Clínic Hospital, 08036 Barcelona, Spain; yblanco@clinic.ub.es
3. Multiple Sclerosis Unit, IRBLLEIDA. Arnau de Vilanova Hospital, 25198 Lleida, Spain; lbrieva.lleida.ics@gencat.cat
4. Multiple Sclerosis and Clinical Neuroimmunology Unit, La Fe Hospital, 46026 Valencia, Spain; Casanova_bon@gva.es
5. Immunology Service, LCMN, Germans Trias University Hospital, 08916 Badalona, Spain; evmcaceres@gmail.com
6. Mellen Center for Multiple Sclerosis, Cleveland Clinic, Cleveland, OH 44195, USA; ontaned@ccf.org
7. Multiple Sclerosis and Neuroimmunology Unit, Dr. Josep Trueta University Hospital and Santa Caterina Hospital, IDIBGI, 17004 Girona, Spain; llramio.girona.ics@gencat.cat
8. Department of Medical Sciences, University of Girona, 17004 Girona, Spain
9. Section of Neuroradiology, Radiology Service, Vall d'Hebron Universitary Hospital, 08035 Barcelona, Spain; alex.rovira.idi@gencat.cat
* Correspondence: cramot.germanstrias@gencat.cat

Abstract: Minimizing the risk of relapse is essential in multiple sclerosis (MS). As none of the treatments currently available are capable of completely preventing relapses, treatment of these episodes remains a cornerstone of MS care. The objective of this manuscript is to reduce uncertainty and improve quality of care of this neurological process. This article addresses definitions of key concepts, recommendations for clinical examination, classification criteria, magnetic resonance imaging, biomarkers, and specific therapeutic counsels including special populations such as pregnant and breastfeeding women, and children. An algorithm for treating MS relapses is also provided.

Keywords: multiple sclerosis; relapse; pseudo-relapses; methylprednisolone; treatment algorithm

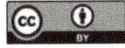

1. Introduction

Multiple sclerosis (MS) is an autoimmune disease of the central nervous system (CNS). It is characterized by inflammation (clinically expressed in the form of relapses), multifocal demyelination, axonal loss, and gliosis in both the white and gray matter. Currently, the cause of MS remains unknown. In experimental autoimmune encephalomyelitis (EAE), an animal model of MS, myelin-specific T cells are believed to play a crucial role in pathogenesis [1]. Much has been published on the role of disease-modifying therapies (DMTs) in reducing annualized relapse rates and relapse severity in MS, but there is comparatively less evidence, or consensus on how relapses should be diagnosed or treated. Early detection and optimal management of relapses will help ensure appropriate control of the disease. A panel of eight experts in the management of MS (the authors) —six neurologists, a neuroradiologist, and an immunologist—was formed to develop this report on the diagnosis and treatment of MS relapses. The aim was to provide a framework to help reduce variability in clinical practice.

2. General Principles

2.1. Relapse

A relapse is the consequence of an immune-mediated attack on the CNS. A patient is suspected of having a relapse when the person reports or is objectively observed to have evidence of a typical acute inflammatory demyelinating event in the central nervous system. Relapses are defined as clinical episodes lasting at least 24 h, in the absence of fever, infection or acute concurrent medical illness [2]. Relapses are also referred to as episodes, bouts, attacks, flares, flare-ups, or exacerbations.

The typical onset of a relapse in MS is subacute with intensity increasing over days, although cases of rapid onset have been described. In most cases, symptoms peak for about 1 to 2 weeks and then typically remit over the next 2 to 4 weeks without treatment. Based on the above time frames, for a relapse to be considered a second distinct event (second episode of CNS inflammatory activity), symptoms must occur at least 30 days after the start of the most recent flare and the new, recurring, or worsening symptoms must last for at least 24 h.

Agreement exists that the appearance of new symptoms within 30 days of initial onset corresponds to worsening of an existing episode, not a new episode. If the symptoms during this period are different to those at onset, the episode is considered to be multifocal. Other conditions, such as spinal cord compression, cerebrovascular disease, pseudo-relapses, and functional syndromes, must always be ruled out when a MS relapse is suspected.

2.2. Pseudo-Relapses

A pseudo-relapse is a clinical episode presenting with signs and symptoms similar to those observed in a previous relapse but in the absence of new inflammatory activity is due to systemic factors that can cause worsening of pre-existing neurologic symptoms. Its onset and resolution typically coincide with the triggering event. The possibility of relapse must be considered in patients whose symptoms persist after resolution of the triggering event or are more severe than prior episodes.

The main triggers of pseudo-relapses are infection (normally urinary or upper respiratory tract), stress, and increased body temperature due to external factors (e.g., a hot shower or high temperatures) or internal factors (e.g., fever or exertion) [3]. Worsening of symptoms caused by an increase in body temperature is known as Uhthoff's phenomenon.

Misdiagnosis of pseudo-relapses often leads to inappropriate corticosteroid treatment or changes to DMT or immunosuppressive therapy, resulting in unnecessary risks and adverse effects.

2.3. Paroxysmal Symptoms

Paroxysmal symptoms are less common manifestations of MS. Paroxysmal symptoms are characterized by their sudden onset, brevity (usually seconds to a few minutes) [4], frequency (from 10 to 20 times per day up to a few hundred times per day), stereotyped fashion, relatively long clinical course (at least 24 h) and typically respond to carbamazepine [5].

Classic paroxysmal symptoms include trigeminal neuralgia, Lhermitte's sign, clusters of tonic spasms, itching, paroxysmal diplopia, paroxysmal dysarthria with ataxia, paroxysmal paresthesia, and paroxysmal hemiparesis or hemitonic spasms. They are not accompanied by altered consciousness or changes in electroencephalographic activity.

When these symptoms occur in isolation, and particularly when they present for the first time, they may be the result of inflammatory activity indicative of a first relapse [6]. If they have occurred previously, they could reflect ephaptic transmission from an existing demyelinating plaque rather than acute disease activity. It is important to recognize and treat them with corticosteroids or carbamazepine as appropriate.

Epileptic seizures, aphasia, and other manifestations of cortical lesions are not considered paroxysmal symptoms in this context.

2.4. Relapse Triggers to Keep in Mind

Relapse rates are higher during the first three months postpartum [7]. Although the evidence is inconclusive, infections [8] including SARS-CoV-2 [9], vaccines [10] and stress [11] may trigger MS relapses too. Withdrawal of an effective DMT [12], monoclonal antibodies targeting tumor necrosis factor alpha (TNF-α) [13], gonadotropin-releasing hormone antagonists (used in the treatment of infertility, hormone-sensitive breast and prostate cancers, certain gynecological disorders and as part of hormone therapy in transgender patients) can also increase the risk of MS relapse [14].

2.5. Relapse Phenotypes

Relapse symptoms are readily identified when they are the result of acute inflammation in the optic nerve, spinal cord or brainstem/cerebellum.

There is increasing evidence that cognitive impairment (e.g., reduced performance at school or work) and psychiatric alterations could be due to an isolated cognitive relapse [15] or non-reactive depression [16]. Therefore it is recommended to quantify all new symptoms using appropriate tests or scales that permit follow-up and comparisons over time.

Relapse presentation tends to be monofocal, but patients can develop multifocal symptoms involving different functional systems as well.

2.6. Relapse Severity

There is currently no validated tool on how to assess the severity of a MS relapse. Physical exam is the most important tool for assessing the severity of MS relapse, the authors stress the importance of using the Expanded Disability Status Scale (EDSS) and recording it in the patient's medical record.

It would be helpful to apply the criteria followed in some clinical trials according to which a relapse can be considered to be mild when there is an EDSS increase of less than 1 point, moderate when there is an increase of 1 to 2.5 points, and severe when there is an increase of 3 or more points [17]. If pre-relapse information is not available in the medical record, a score of 2 or higher in the visual, brainstem, or pyramidal functional systems is required for optic neuritis, myelitis, or brainstem relapse respectively. In the case of relapse in an uncertain location, a score of at least 2 points in the EDSS is necessary [18,19].

The authors consider that it is important to quantify the severity and apply the proposed therapeutic algorithm (Figure 1) until more evidence is available. In this way, the EDSS at the time of relapse can be compared with the previous EDSS allowing to quantify the increase in disability related to the relapse (EDSS score on relapse minus previous EDSS score).

2.7. Relapse Recovery

Remission is not a synonym of recovery. Recovery is considered to occur when the patient's disability levels return to pre-relapse levels. Patients who do not recover pre-relapse function and disability levels (measured by EDSS) within 6 months of treatment are considered to usually have permanent sequelae.

Some authors have postulated that severe relapses and longer duration are associated with a greater risk of sequelae [20]. There is some evidence that recovery after 12 weeks of treatment with methylprednisolone (MP) is determined by pre-relapse EDSS scores rather than relapse severity, with lower remission rates observed in patients with a pre-relapse score of over 3.0 [21].

3. Clinical Examination

The author's recommendations for the evaluation of patients in relapse are summarized in Table 1.

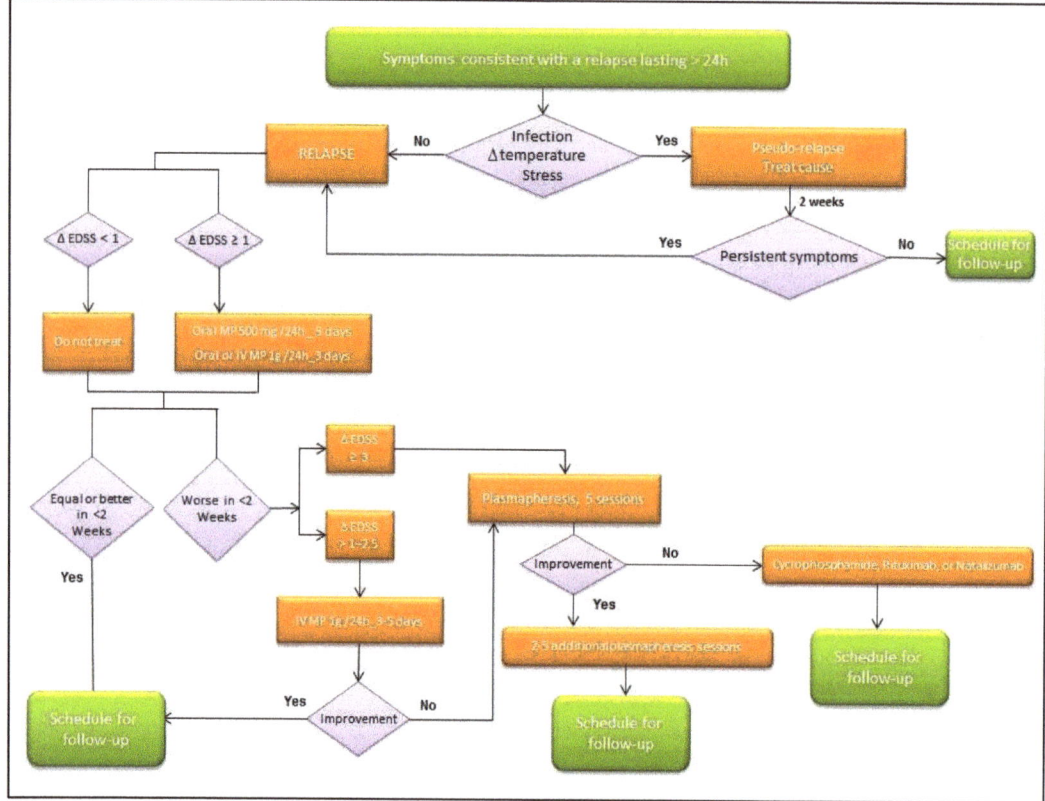

Figure 1. Therapeutic algorithm of MS relapse.

Table 1. Recommendations for the Assessment of Patients with Suspected Relapse.

Recommendations for the Assessment of Patients with Suspected Relapse
Mandatory: - Date of onset   - Clinical topography and if monofocal or multifocal   - Visual acuity measured using a Snellen chart   - Visual contrast sensitivity test in patients with optic neuritis   - Functional system scores   - EDSS score   - Re-evaluate patients by telephone or electronic communication after 2 weeks and instruct them to contact a provider if they notice worsening of symptoms   - Follow-up visit at 6 months
Optional: - Symbol Digit Modalities Test (SDMT)   - Nine-hole peg test (9HPT)   - Timed 25-foot walk test (T25FW) (7.62 m)

4. Treatment

The treatment goals for patients with a MS relapse are to shorten the duration and severity of the episode, relieve symptoms and increase recovery.

4.1. Which Types of Relapse Should Be Treated?

Corticosteroids relieve and shorten the duration of relapse symptoms but do not prevent sequelae and do not modify the disease course of MS over time [22]. It is therefore recommended not to treat mild relapses (increase in EDSS < 1 point), sensory relapses in particular, unless they have a significant impact on quality of life, and unless the potential benefits of treatment outweigh the potential adverse effects (AEs). Patients with remitting symptoms are often not treated.

4.2. Therapeutic Window

Patients should be made aware of the importance of informing their MS specialist team as soon as they suspect a relapse to ensure prompt evaluation, exclusion of a pseudo-relapse, and initiation of high-dose corticosteroids where appropriate.

4.3. Corticosteroid Treatment

The standard first-line treatment for relapses is corticosteroid therapy using high-doses of methylprednisolone (MP). The UK NICE (National Institute for Health and Care Excellence) guidelines [23] recommend administering at least 500 mg of oral MP every 24 h for 5 consecutive days. An alternative is to recommend 1 g of oral MP for 3 to 5 consecutive days [18,24,25] even for optic neuritis [26] given scientific evidence available to date.

The oral formulation offers greater convenience: enables treatment during weekends, prevents the patient from having to go to an outpatient clinic (a significant advantage during the SARS-COVID-19 pandemic) and results in considerable savings in terms of healthcare costs and prevents work productivity loss. As the vast majority of countries do not have access to oral commercial formulations of high-dose MP, hospital pharmacies need to prepare these formulations or request the manufacturers to produce tablets of various doses. Ideally, patients should be prescribed 500 mg tablets to enable the administration of 500-mg/24 h for 5 consecutive days or 1000 (500 + 500) mg/24 h for 3–5 consecutive days. The US Food and Drug Administration (FDA) or the European Medicines Agency (EMA) have not approved MP for oral use.

1 g of intravenous MP for 3 to 5 consecutive days can be administered if preferred by the physician or patient, in cases where oral MP has failed or is not tolerated, and if hospitalization is required due to severe symptoms, or to monitor other medical or psychological conditions such as diabetes and depression.

There is evidence suggesting that tapering doses of oral corticosteroids following high-dose administration does not offer benefits [27] and there is no significant risk of adrenal suppression.

Patients must be informed that they should expect to see an improvement within an average of 1 to 2 weeks of starting the first course of MP.

Patients with moderate relapses who do not tolerate MP could be candidates for adrenocorticotropic hormone therapy [28] administered as an intramuscular or subcutaneous injection at 80–120 units for 14–21 days. A growing number of studies report favorable results in this setting. However, ACTH gel is significantly more expensive than steroids.

4.4. Inadequate Response to MP

The authors agreed that the definition of inadequate treatment response included worsening of the EDSS within 2 weeks of MP initiation. If the increase in EDSS is moderate (1–2.5 points), a second course of MP should be given as per the recommendations in the section on corticosteroid treatment. If the increase is substantial ($\geq$3 points), treatment with plasmapheresis should contemplated. Plasmapheresis is the only second-line treatment for steroid-resistant exacerbations supported by solid clinical evidence [29]. The procedure is performed every other day to reach a total of five sessions, although a shorter may be used in patients showing an optimal response.

Patients with a suboptimal response after five plasmapheresis exchanges or patients in whom MRI shows persistent acute inflammatory activity should be started on a third-line therapy. Options include (1) cytotoxic therapy with myeloablative agents such as cyclophosphamide (200 mg/kg/d for 4 days intravenously) [30], or (2) an initial high loading dose of rituximab (2000 mg intravenously) divided into 2 infusions given 2 weeks apart to attack antibody-secreting B lymphocytes [31], or (3) a single dose of natalizumab (300 mg intravenously) to prevent lymphocytes from crossing the blood-brain barrier [32]. These third-line treatments, which can also be used for fulminant or tumefactive demyelination, are not supported by strong evidence, but are commonly used in severe cases.

Data suggest that intravenous immunoglobulin therapy is not useful [32–34], but it could be a suitable option for patients with severe relapses who do not have access to a center with plasmapheresis.

Patients with severe relapses who are intolerant to MP should be treated with plasmapheresis.

4.5. Adverse Effects of Methylprednisolone

Patients must be warned that they may experience immediate adverse effects (AEs) during treatment with high-dose MP. AEs are generally mild or moderate. The most common AEs are insomnia, mood changes (irritability, euphoria and depression), gastrointestinal disorders, palpitations, weight gain, edema, acne, headache, musculoskeletal pain, and a metallic taste in the mouth. Patients should also be warned about the risk of infections, such as herpes, sepsis, pneumonia, arthritis, bursitis, and complicated urinary infections.

The need for prophylactic treatment of AEs should be assessed on a case-by-case basis. Examples are insomnia medication and gastroprotective drugs for patients with a history of peptic ulcers, acid reflux, or hiatal hernia. Diabetic patients should be advised to monitor their blood sugar levels closely, and despite the lack of evidence, non-diabetic patients should undergo capillary blood glucose testing at their primary care center or local pharmacy. Blood pressure should also be monitored in patients with hypertension.

Serious events are rare. The most common serious event are psychosis, depression, and mania. There have been very few reports of reactivation of latent infections to date, but caution is warranted as patients on immunosuppressive DMT are at an increased risk. There are no data showing that high-dose MP significantly increases the risk of latent chronic infections.

High doses of MP are considered to be immunosuppressive. MP should not be administered 8 weeks before or 8 weeks after the administration of live or attenuated live vaccines because of the increased risk of complications due to viral replication [35]. Vaccines containing inactivated or killed organisms may be used, although response may be diminished.

4.6. Symptomatic Treatment during MS Relapses

It should be contemplated for pain, spasticity, and diminished sphincter control, as it can improve function, patient comfort, and quality of life.

The benefits of rehabilitation during acute relapse are not well established [36] but in general is recommended. Patients with fatigue and motor or sensory cord deficits may need to rest and be warned about the risk of falls, while those with sensory deficits for pain should be warned of the risk of injury.

4.7. Relapse Treatment during Pregnancy

The FDA does not classify MP as a pregnancy risk drug.

High-dose corticosteroids administered for short periods (3–5 days) appear to be safe during pregnancy, especially in the second and third trimesters.

There is conflicting evidence on the association between corticosteroid use during pregnancy and the risk of cleft lip and/or cleft palate [37]. There is little evidence that systemic corticosteroid use in pregnancy independently increases the risk of preterm birth, low birth weight, or preeclampsia. Currently, there is not enough evidence to determine whether systemic corticosteroids might contribute to gestational diabetes mellitus [38].

Intravenous immunoglobulins could be a suitable option for patients with severe relapses who do not respond to MP, although the risk of AEs such as cerebral venous thrombosis (which has an increased risk of occurring during pregnancy) must be contemplated [39]. Plasmapheresis performed under expert supervision can also be considered in such cases. The couple must always be involved in treatment decisions.

4.8. Relapse Treatment during Breastfeeding

Women with MS are at an increased risk of relapse in the postpartum period. Although the level of MP transfer into breast milk is very low, generally IVMP treatment is not advised during breastfeeding. If the mother wishes to continue breastfeeding, intravenous MP is preferable to oral, as it has a shorter peak effect. Patients should wait for 2–4 h before breastfeeding after administration of MP, as there is evidence that levels in infants after this time are lower than those in infants being treated with MP for another condition (0.25 mg/kg) [40]. Another option is to breastfeed only before receiving high doses of MP. Mothers can also use the approach of expressing milk using a breast pump, which can later be offered to the baby, before receiving MP.

4.9. Relapse Treatment in Children

Considering the lack of evidence regarding the treatment of MS relapses in the pediatric population, the recommendations in children are based on data from adult studies. MP is the most commonly selected first-line therapy for disabling MS relapses in children. The recommended treatment is intravenous MP 30 mg/kg/d (maximum 1000 mg/d) for 3–5 consecutive days [41]. Although equivalent studies have not been performed in children, it is assumed that high-dose oral corticosteroids will be similarly effective for the treatment of MS relapses in children and adults. Oral corticosteroid taper for the treatment of relapses is not a routine practice in pediatric MS. One exception is acute disseminated encephalomyelitis, where the recommended treatment is high-dose corticosteroids followed by an oral taper over 4–6 weeks with a starting dose of prednisone of 1–2 mg/kg/day. A taper period of 4–6 weeks is recommended as an increased risk of relapse has been observed with periods of 3 weeks or less [42].

As with adults, non-responders should be administered a second course of MP or treated with plasmapheresis [43].

The author's algorithm for treating MS relapses is summarized in Figure 1.

4.10. Treatment of Asymptomatic Active Lesions on MRI

It is difficult to evaluate the immediate or delayed effects of treatment initiated for acute lesions without clinical correlates. Magnetic resonance Imaging (MRI) studies have shown that focal signal abnormalities reflecting inflammatory activity can precede clinical manifestations by several weeks [44]. Because of this mismatch between imaging and clinical manifestations, it is possible that by the time a patient develops symptoms and is prescribed corticosteroid treatment, he or she may already have developed permanent residual disability due to demyelination and even axonal damage. There are neurologists who think that an asymptomatic new lesion on MRI should be treated accordingly [45] and others who think otherwise, as there is no evidence of the comparative effectiveness of these approaches [46,47].

There is also no evidence available on whether or not to treat large or numerous asymptomatic lesions involving the brainstem or spinal cord.

The authors recommend performing a more exhaustive examination (using the SDMT, the Nine-Hole Peg Test, or a fatigue scale) in patients with "asymptomatic" active lesions detected by MRI to establish whether lesions are truly subclinical.

5. MRI Studies during Relapses

MRI is the gold standard diagnostic test for MS but it is often impractical to obtain in a timely fashion in relation to relapse and can miss lesions for determined variety of reasons. Brain and spinal cord MRI scans are not necessary in patients with a clear diagnosis of MS relapse. They are, however, recommended in patients with an unclear or non-objectively observed clinical relapse and should be performed before starting corticosteroid treatment, as corticosteroids can reduce the time during which lesions show contrast uptake. MRI should be performed ideally within the first 72 h if steroid treatment is planned, and within 2 to 3 weeks of relapse onset in patients that do not receive steroid treatment because mean enhancement duration without treatment is 2–4 weeks [48].

A brain MRI study can demonstrate gadolinium-enhancing lesions when cognitive impairment, depression, or even excessive fatigue is suspected to be due to a new episode of inflammatory activity.

Sometimes a spinal cord MRI is deemed necessary to confirm a relapse likely related to spinal cord involvement. A brain MRI is also necessary in such cases, as active spinal lesions tend to be associated with active cerebral lesions, which are easier to identify. This combined strategy increases the likelihood of detecting active inflammatory lesions. However, adding spinal cord MRI to brain MRI in patients with relapses related to brain lesions does not appear to increase the sensitivity of MRI for detecting disease activity.

The abbreviated MAGNIMS (Magnetic Resonance Imaging in MS) MRI protocol should be followed at all times [49,50]. The contrast agent should be injected at least 5, and ideally 10, minutes before obtaining the T1 sequence. This wait time can be used to obtain other sequences included in the protocol (T2-FLAIR, T2).

MRI studies, particularly MRI conducted with contrast, should be avoided during the first trimester of pregnancy.

The author's recommendations for the MRI assessment of patients in relapse are summarized in Table 2.

Table 2. Recommendations for the MRI Assessment of Patients with Suspected Relapse.

Recommendations for the MRI Assessment of Patients with Suspected Relapse
- Obtain MRI for diagnostic and prognostic purposes during the first relapse (clinically isolated syndrome)
- Obtain MRI before treatment escalation in patients who do not respond to corticosteroids
- Obtain MRI before treatment initiation with corticosteroids in patients with severe, unexpected relapses
- Obtain MRI in patients with an unclear or non-objectively observed clinical diagnosis
- Obtain MRI in patients in whom gadolinium-enhanced lesions must be demonstrated before initiation of immunomodulatory treatment.

6. Biomarkers

There have been reports of changes in lymphocyte subpopulations that can predict or support the occurrence of a relapse and that normalize after corticosteroid treatment [51,52]. There are, however, no immune related biomarkers currently available outside research applications.

Neurofilament light (NfL) chain protein is a cytoskeletal protein located in neuronal axons. Increased cerebrospinal fluid and blood NfL levels have been described in MS (following axonal injury) and other diseases. They have also been linked to aging. The possible value of NfL as a biomarker for MS relapses has been postulated in recent years, as increased levels have been associated with the presence of gadolinium-enhancing lesions on MRI [53]. In this context, in patients with early MS, the presence of both abnormal NfL and thin ganglion cell and inner plexiform layer in retinal optical coherence tomography (OCT) have been described as additive risk factors of disease activity [54].

More recently, wide metabolomic studies have shown metabolic perturbations during relapses, and several serum metabolites, mainly lysine and asparagine (higher in relapses), as well as isoleucine and leucine (lower in relapses), postulated as potential biomarkers useful to differentiate relapse from remission. Future metabolomics studies will need to prospectively include MRI scans to understand metabolic signatures and their relation with MRI-defined inflammation [55].

7. Conclusions

Diagnosis and particularly treatment of MS relapses varies greatly among clinicians. This document offers a series of simple and practical statements with recommendations that, although not reaching full consensus,, reflect the realities of current clinical practice. They are easy to implement in daily practice and can be readily adapted to the specific needs of practitioners seeking to standardize care processes in MS. Further studies on larger cohorts are required to confirm the effectiveness of the interventions regarding relapses in MS.

Author Contributions: Conceptualization, C.R.-T.; Validation, C.R.-T.; Visualization, Y.B., LB, B.C., E.M.-C., D.O., L.R.-T. and À.R.; Writing—original draft, C.R.-T.; Writing—review & editing, C.R.-T., Y.B., L.B., B.C., E.M.-C., D.O., L.R.-T. and À.R. All authors have read and agreed to the published version of the manuscript.

Funding: This research was funded by NOVARTIS FARMACÉUTICA, SA, for the two expert panel meetings held and the recording and transcription of the content of the first meeting performed by the contract research organization, Dynamic.

Institutional Review Board Statement: Not applicable.

Informed Consent Statement: Not applicable.

Data Availability Statement: Not applicable.

Acknowledgments: The authors would like to thank Praneeta Raza and Susi Soler for editorial assistance with the manuscript.

Conflicts of Interest: Cristina Ramo-Tello has received personal compensation for scientific consultancy work and/or help with travel expenses for attending conferences from Biogen Idec, Merck Serono, Novartis, Sanofi-Genzyme, Almirall, Brystol and Roche. The Institut d'Investigació en Ciències de la Salut Germans Trias i Pujol, where Ramo-Tello works has received grants from Novartis, Sanofi-Genzyme, Bristol, Roche and Almirall. Yolanda Blanco has received speaker honoraria from Novartis, Roche, Merck, Genzyme-Sanofi and Biogen. Luis Brieva has received support for research projects from his group as well as speakers' and consultancy fees and help with travel expenses for attending conferences from Bayer, Biogen, Roche, Merk, Novartis, Allmirall, and Sanofi. B. Casanova serves on scientific advisory boards for Novartis, Sanofi-Genzyme, and Roche, and has received speaker honoraria from Sanofi-Genzyme, Merck-Serono, Teva Pharmaceutical Industries Ltd., Novartis, Roche, Celgene and Biogen. Eva Martinez-Cáceres has received personal compensation for scientific consultancy, speaker honoraria or help with travel expenses for attending conferences from Biogen Idec, Merck Serono, Novartis, Sanofi-Genzyme and Roche. D. Ontaneda has received research support from National Multiple Sclerosis Society, National Institutes of Health, Patient Centered Outcomes Research Institute, Race to Erase MS Foundation, Genentech, and Genzyme. He has also received consulting fees from Biogen, Genentech/Roche, Genzyme, and Merck. Ll. Ramió serves on scientific advisory boards for Novartis, Sanofi-Genzyme, Roche, Celgene and Almirall, and has received speaker honoraria from Roche, Biogen, Novartis, Sanofi-Genzyme, Merck, Celgene, Bayer and Teva Pharmaceutical Industries Ltd. Rovira serves on scientific advisory boards for Novartis, Sanofi-Genzyme, SyntheticMR, Bayer, Roche, Biogen, and OLEA Medical, and has received speaker honoraria from Bayer, Sanofi-Genzyme, Bracco, Merck-Serono, Teva Pharmaceutical Industries Ltd., Novartis, Roche and Biogen. The funders had no role in the writing of the manuscript, or in the decision to publish it. The authors confirm that this manuscript complies with ethical standards.

References

1. Mansilla, M.J.; Presas-Rodríguez, S.; Teniente-Serra, A.; González-Larreategui, I.; Quirant-Sánchez, B.; Fondelli, F.; Djedovic, N.; Iwaszkiewicz-Grześ, D.; Chwojnicki, K.; Miljković, Đ.; et al. Paving the way towards an effective treatment for multiple sclerosis: Advances in cell therapy. *Cell. Mol. Immunol.* **2021**, *18*, 1353–1374. [CrossRef]
2. Polman, C.H.; Reingold, S.C.; Banwell, B.; Clanet, M.; Cohen, J.A.; Filippi, M.; Fujihara, K.; Havrdova, E.; Hutchinson, M.; Kappos, L.; et al. Diagnostic criteria for multiple sclerosis: 2010 Revisions to the McDonald criteria. *Ann. Neurol.* **2011**, *69*, 292–302. [CrossRef]
3. Keegan, B.M. *Multiple Sclerosis Clinician's Guide to Diagnosis and Treatment*; Birnbaum, G., Ed.; Oxford University Press: Oxford, UK, 2013; ISBN-13: 978-0199840786.
4. Ehling, R.; Bsteh, G.; Di Pauli, F.; Hegen, H.; Auer, M.; Obermair, K.; Wagner, M.; Deisenhammer, F.; Reindl, M.; Berger, T. Rethinking the importance of paroxysmal and unusual symptoms as first clinical manifestation of multiple sclerosis: They do matter. *Mult. Scler. Relat. Disord.* **2016**, *9*, 150–154. [CrossRef] [PubMed]
5. Tüzün, E.; Akman-Demir, G.; Eraksoy, M. Paroxysmal attacks in multiple sclerosis. *Mult. Scler. J.* **2001**, *7*, 402–404. [CrossRef] [PubMed]
6. Matthews, W.B. Paroxysmal symptoms in multiple sclerosis. *J. Neurol. Neurosurg. Psychiatry* **1975**, *38*, 617–623. [CrossRef]
7. Confavreux, C.; Hutchinson, M.; Hours, M.M.; Cortinovis-Tourniaire, P.; Moreau, T. Rate of Pregnancy-Related Relapse in Multiple Sclerosis. *N. Engl. J. Med.* **1998**, *339*, 285–291. [CrossRef]
8. Andersen, O.; Lygner, P.-E.; Andersson, M.; Vablne, A. Viral infections trigger multiple sclerosis relapses: A prospective seroepidemiological study. *J. Neurol.* **1993**, *240*, 417–422. [CrossRef]
9. Etemadifar, M.; Sedaghat, N.; Aghababaee, A.; Kargaran, P.K.; Maracy, M.R.; Ganjalikhani-Hakemi, M.; Rayani, M.; Abhari, A.P.; Khorvash, R.; Salari, M.; et al. COVID-19 and the Risk of Relapse in Multiple Sclerosis Patients: A Fight with No Bystander Effect? *Mult. Scler. Relat. Disord.* **2021**, *51*, 102915. [CrossRef]
10. Confavreux, C.; Suissa, S.; Saddier, P.; Bourdès, V.; Vukusic, S. Vaccinations and the Risk of Relapse in Multiple Sclerosis. *N. Engl. J. Med.* **2001**, *344*, 319–326. [CrossRef]
11. Mohr, D.C.; Lovera, J.; Brown, T.; Cohen, B.; Neylan, T.; Henry, R.; Siddique, J.; Jin, L.; Daikh, D.; Pelletier, D. A randomized trial of stress management for the prevention of new brain lesions in MS. *Neurology* **2012**, *79*, 412–419. [CrossRef] [PubMed]
12. Berkovich, R. Clinical and MRI outcomes after stopping or switching disease-modifying therapy in stable MS patients: A case series report. *Mult. Scler. Relat. Disord.* **2017**, *17*, 123–127. [CrossRef]
13. Kemanetzoglou, E.; Andreadou, E. CNS Demyelination with TNF-α Blockers. *Curr. Neurol. Neurosci. Rep.* **2017**, *17*, 36. [CrossRef] [PubMed]
14. Correale, J.; Farez, M.F.; Ysrraelit, M.C. Increase in multiple sclerosis activity after assisted reproduction technology. *Ann. Neurol.* **2012**, *72*, 682–694. [CrossRef]
15. Pardini, M.; Uccelli, A.; Grafman, J.; Özgür, Y.; Mancardi, G.; Roccatagliata, L. Isolated cognitive relapses in multiple sclerosis. *J. Neurol. Neurosurg. Psychiatry* **2014**, *85*, 1035–1037. [CrossRef]
16. Butler, C.; Zeman, A.Z. Neurological syndromes which can be mistaken for psychiatric conditions. *J. Neurol. Neurosurg. Psychiatry* **2005**, *76*, i31–i38. [CrossRef]
17. Nos, C.; Garriga, J.S.; Borràs, C.; Rio, J.; Tintore, M.; Montalban, X. Clinical impact of intravenous methylprednisolone in attacks of multiple sclerosis. *Mult. Scler. J.* **2004**, *10*, 413–416. [CrossRef]
18. Ramo-Tello, C.; Grau-López, L.; Tintoré, M.; Rovira, A.; Torrenta, L.R.I.; Brieva, L.; Cano, A.; Carmona, O.; Saiz, A.; Torres, F.; et al. A randomized clinical trial of oral versus intravenous methylprednisolone for relapse of MS. *Mult. Scler. J.* **2014**, *20*, 717–725. [CrossRef]
19. Hervás-García, J.V.; Ramió-Torrentà, L.; Brieva-Ruiz, L.; Batllé-Nadal, J.; Moral, E.; Blanco, Y.; Cano-Orgaz, A.; Presas-Rodríguez, S.; Torres, F.; Capellades, J.; et al. Comparison of two high doses of oral methylprednisolone for multiple sclerosis relapses: A pilot, multicentre, randomized, double-blind, non-inferiority trial. *Eur. J. Neurol.* **2019**, *26*, 525–532. [CrossRef] [PubMed]
20. Hirst, C.L.; Ingram, G.; Pickersgill, T.P.; Robertson, N.P. Temporal evolution of remission following multiple sclerosis relapse and predictors of outcome. *Mult. Scler. J.* **2012**, *18*, 1152–1158. [CrossRef]
21. Ramo-Tello, C.; Tintoré, M.; Rovira, A.; Ramió-Torrenta, L.; Brieva, L.; Saiz, A.; Cano, A.; Carmona, O.; Hervás, J.V.; Grau-López, L. Baseline clinical status as a predictor of methylprednisolone response in multiple sclerosis relapses. *Mult. Scler. J.* **2016**, *22*, 117–121. [CrossRef] [PubMed]
22. Brusaferri, F.; Candelise, L. Steriods for multiple sclerosis and optic neuritis: A meta-analysis of randomized controlled clinical trials. *J. Neurol.* **2000**, *247*, 435–442. [CrossRef] [PubMed]
23. National Clinical Guideline Centre (UK). *Multiple Sclerosis: Management of Multiple Sclerosis in Primary and Secondary Care*; National Institute for Health and Care Excellence: London, UK, 2014.
24. Burton, J.M.; O'Connor, P.W.; Hohol, M.; Beyene, J. Oral versus intravenous steroids for treatment of relapses in multiple sclerosis. *Cochrane Database Syst. Rev.* **2012**, *12*, CD006921. [CrossRef] [PubMed]
25. Le Page, E.; Veillard, D.; Laplaud, D.; Hamonic, S.; Wardi, R.; Lebrun-Frenay, C.; Zagnoli, F.; Wiertlewski, S.; Deburghgraeve, V.; Coustans, M.; et al. Oral versus intravenous high-dose methylprednisolone for treatment of relapses in patients with multiple sclerosis (COPOUSEP): A randomised, controlled, double-blind, non-inferiority trial. *Lancet* **2015**, *386*, 974–981. [CrossRef]

26. Morrow, S.A.; Fraser, J.A.; Day, C.; Bowman, D.; Rosehart, H.; Kremenchutzky, M.; Nicolle, M. Effect of Treating Acute Optic Neuritis with Bioequivalent Oral vs Intravenous Corticosteroids. *JAMA Neurol.* **2018**, *75*, 690–696. [CrossRef]
27. Perumal, J.S.; Caon, C.; Hreha, S.; Zabad, R.; Tselis, A.; Lisak, R.; Khan, O. Oral prednisone taper following intravenous steroids fails to improve disability or recovery from relapses in multiple sclerosis. *Eur. J. Neurol.* **2008**, *15*, 677–680. [CrossRef]
28. Rose, A.S.; Kuzma, J.W.; Kurtzke, J.F.; Namerow, N.S.; Sibley, W.A.; Tourtellotte, W.W. Cooperative study in the evaluation of therapy in multiple sclerosis: ACTH vs. placebo final report. *Neurology* **1970**, *20*, 1–59. [CrossRef]
29. Cortese, I.; Chaudhry, V.; So, Y.T.; Cantor, F.; Cornblath, D.R.; Rae-Grant, A. Evidence-based guideline update: Plasmapheresis in neurologic disorders: Report of the Therapeutics and Technology Assessment Subcommittee of the American Academy of Neurology. *Neurology* **2011**, *76*, 294–300. [CrossRef]
30. Harrison, D.M.; Gladstone, D.E.; Hammond, E.; Cheng, J.; Jones, R.J.; Brodsky, R.A.; Kerr, D.; McArthur, J.C.; Kaplin, A. Treatment of relapsing–remitting multiple sclerosis with high-dose cyclophosphamide induction followed by glatiramer acetate maintenance. *Mult. Scler. J.* **2012**, *18*, 202–209. [CrossRef] [PubMed]
31. Yamout, B.I.; El-Ayoubi, N.K.; Nicolas, J.; El Kouzi, Y.; Khoury, S.J.; Zeineddine, M.M. Safety and Efficacy of Rituximab in Multiple Sclerosis: A Retrospective Observational Study. *J. Immunol. Res.* **2018**, *2018*, 9084759. [CrossRef]
32. O'Connor, P.W.; Goodman, A.; Willmer-Hulme, A.J.; Libonati, M.A.; Metz, L.; Murray, R.S.; Sheremata, W.A.; Vollmer, T.L.; Stone, L.A.; the Natalizumab Multiple Sclerosis Trial Group. Randomized multicenter trial of natalizumab in acute MS relapses: Clinical and MRI effects. *Neurology* **2004**, *62*, 2038–2043. [CrossRef]
33. Fazekas, F.; Lublin, F.D.; Li, D.; Freedman, M.S.; Hartung, H.P.; Rieckmann, P.; Sorensen, P.S.; Maas-Enriquez, M.; Sommerauer, B.; Hanna, K.; et al. Intravenous immunoglobulin in relapsing-remitting multiple sclerosis: A dose-finding trial. *Neurology* **2008**, *71*, 265–271. [CrossRef]
34. Noseworthy, J.H.; O'Brien, P.C.; Petterson, T.M.; Weis, J.; Stevens, L.; Peterson, W.K.; Sneve, D.; Cross, S.A.; Leavitt, J.A.; Auger, R.G.; et al. A randomized trial of intravenous immunoglobulin in inflammatory demyelinating optic neuritis. *Neurology* **2001**, *56*, 1514–1522. [CrossRef] [PubMed]
35. Immunization Action Coalition. Available online: https://www.immunize.org/askexperts/contraindications-precautions.asp (accessed on 30 November 2019).
36. Asano, M.; Raszewski, R.; Finlayson, M. Rehabilitation Interventions for the Management of Multiple Sclerosis Relapse. *Int. J. MS Care* **2014**, *16*, 99–104. [CrossRef]
37. Carmichael, S.L.; Shaw, G.M. Maternal corticosteroid use and risk of selected congenital anomalies. *Am. J. Med. Genet.* **1999**, *86*, 242–244. [CrossRef]
38. Bandoli, G.; Palmsten, K.; Smith, C.J.F.; Chambers, C.D. A Review of Systemic Corticosteroid Use in Pregnancy and the Risk of Select Pregnancy and Birth Outcomes. *Rheum. Dis. Clin. N. Am.* **2017**, *43*, 489–502. [CrossRef]
39. Haas, J.; Hommes, O.R. A dose comparison study of IVIG in postpartum relapsing-remitting multiple sclerosis. *Mult. Scler. J.* **2007**, *13*, 900–908. [CrossRef] [PubMed]
40. Boz, C.; Terzi, M.; Karahan, S.Z.; Sen, S.; Sarac, Y.; Mavis, M.E. Safety of IV pulse methylprednisolone therapy during breastfeeding in patients with multiple sclerosis. *Mult. Scler. J.* **2018**, *24*, 1205–1211. [CrossRef]
41. Wilbur, C.; Yeh, E.A. Improving Outcomes in Pediatric Multiple Sclerosis: Current and Emerging Treatments. *Pediatr. Drugs* **2019**, *21*, 137–152. [CrossRef] [PubMed]
42. Dale, R.C.; De Sousa, C.; Chong, W.K.; Cox, T.C.S.; Harding, B.; Neville, B.G.R. Acute disseminated encephalomyelitis, multiphasic disseminated encephalomyelitis and multiple sclerosis in children. *Brain* **2000**, *123*, 2407–2422. [CrossRef]
43. Bigi, S.; Banwell, B.; Yeh, E.A. Outcomes After Early Administration of Plasma Exchange in Pediatric Central Nervous System Inflammatory Demyelination. *J. Child Neurol.* **2015**, *30*, 874–880. [CrossRef]
44. Barkhof, F.; Scheltens, P.; Frequin, S.T.; Nauta, J.J.; Tas, M.W.; Valk, J.; Hommes, O.R. Relapsing-remitting multiple sclerosis: Sequential enhanced MR imaging vs clinical findings in determining disease activity. *Am. J. Roentgenol.* **1992**, *159*, 1041–1047. [CrossRef] [PubMed]
45. Rojas, J.I.; Patrucco, L.; Cristiano, E. An asymptomatic new lesion on MRI is a relapse and should be treated accordingly—Yes. *Mult. Scler. J.* **2019**, *25*, 1842–1843. [CrossRef]
46. Chard, D.T.; Trip, S.A. An asymptomatic new lesion on MRI is a relapse and should be treated accordingly—No. *Mult. Scler. J.* **2019**, *25*, 1843–1845. [CrossRef]
47. Arrambide, G.; Tintore, M. An asymptomatic new lesion on MRI is a relapse and should be treated accordingly—Commentary. *Mult. Scler. J.* **2019**, *25*, 1845–1847. [CrossRef]
48. Cotton, F.; Weiner, H.L.; Jolesz, F.A.; Guttmann, C. MRI contrast uptake in new lesions in relapsing-remitting MS followed at weekly intervals. *Neurology* **2003**, *60*, 640–646. [CrossRef]
49. Rovira, À.; Wattjes, M.P.; Tintoré, M.; Tur, C.; Yousry, T.A.; Sormani, M.P.; De Stefano, N.; Filippi, M.; Auger, C.; MAGNIMS Study Group; et al. MAGNIMS study group. Evidence-based guidelines: MAGNIMS consensus guidelines on the use of MRI in multiple sclerosis-clinical implementation in the diagnostic process. *Nat. Rev. Neurol.* **2015**, *8*, 471–482. [CrossRef]
50. Wattjes, M.P.; Rovira, À.; Miller, D.; Yousry, T.A.; Sormani, M.P.; de Stefano, N.; Tintoré, M.; Auger, C.; Tur, C.; MAGNIMS Study Group. Evidence-based guidelines: MAGNIMS consensus guidelines on the use of MRI in multiple sclerosis—Establishing disease prognosis and monitoring patients. *Nat. Rev. Neurol.* **2015**, *11*, 597–606. [CrossRef]

51. Liu, M.; Hu, X.; Wang, Y.; Peng, F.; Yang, Y.; Chen, X.; Lu, Z.; Zheng, X. Effect of high-dose methylprednisolone treatment on Th17 cells in patients with multiple sclerosis in relapse. *Acta Neurol. Scand.* **2009**, *120*, 235–241. [CrossRef]
52. Martínez-Cáceres, E.M.; Barrau, M.A.; Brieva, L.; Espejo, C.; Barberà, N.; Montalban, X. Treatment with methylprednisolone in relapses of multiple sclerosis patients: Immunological evidence of immediate and short-term but not long-lasting effects. *Clin. Exp. Immunol.* **2002**, *127*, 165–171. [CrossRef] [PubMed]
53. Varhaug, K.N.; Barro, C.; Bjørnevik, K.; Myhr, K.-M.; Torkildsen, Ø.; Wergeland, S.; Bindoff, L.A.; Kuhle, J.; Vedeler, C. Neurofilament light chain predicts disease activity in relapsing-remitting MS. *Neurol. Neuroimmunol. Neuroinflamm.* **2017**, *5*, e422. [CrossRef] [PubMed]
54. Lin, T.-Y.; Vitkova, V.; Asseyer, S.; Serra, I.M.; Motamedi, S.; Chien, C.; Ditzhaus, M.; Papadopoulou, A.; Benkert, P.; Kuhle, J.; et al. Increased Serum Neurofilament Light and Thin Ganglion Cell–Inner Plexiform Layer Are Additive Risk Factors for Disease Activity in Early Multiple Sclerosis. *Neurol. Neuroimmunol. Neuroinflamm.* **2021**, *8*, e1051. [CrossRef] [PubMed]
55. Yeo, T.; Probert, F.; Sealey, M.; Saldana, L.; Geraldes, R.; Höeckner, S.; Schiffer, E.; Claridge, T.D.W.; Leppert, D.; DeLuca, G.; et al. Objective Biomarkers for Clinical Relapse in Multiple Sclerosis: A Metabolomics Approach. *Brain Commun.* **2021**, *3*, fcab240. [CrossRef] [PubMed]

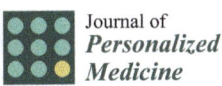

Review

Escalation vs. Early Intense Therapy in Multiple Sclerosis

Bonaventura Casanova [1,*], Carlos Quintanilla-Bordás [1] and Francisco Gascón [2]

1 Unitat de Neuroimmunologia, Hospital Universitari i Politècnic La Fe. València, la Universitat de València, 46026 Valencia, Spain; carlosqb@gmail.com
2 Unitat de Neuroimmunologia, Hospital Clínic Universitari de València, 46010 Valencia, Spain; kokogascon@hotmail.com
* Correspondence: casanova.bonaventura@gmail.com

Abstract: The treatment strategy of multiple sclerosis (MS) is a highly controversial debate. Currently, there are up to 19 drugs approved. However, there is no clear evidence to guide fundamental decisions such as what treatment should be chosen in first place, when treatment failure or suboptimal response should be considered, or what treatment should be considered in these cases. The "escalation strategy" consists of starting treatment with drugs of low side-effect profile and low efficacy, and "escalating" to drugs of higher efficacy—with more potential side-effects—if necessary. This strategy has prevailed over the years. However, the evidence supporting this strategy is based on short-term studies, in hope that the benefits will stand in the long term. These studies usually do not consider the heterogeneity of the disease and the limited effect that relapses have on the long-term. On the other hand, "early intense therapy" strategy refers to starting treatment with drugs of higher efficacy from the beginning, despite having a less favorable side-effect profile. This approach takes advantage of the so-called "window of opportunity" in hope to maximize the clinical benefits in the long-term. At present, the debate remains open. In this review, we will critically review both strategies. We provide a summary of the current evidence for each strategy without aiming to reach a definite conclusion.

Keywords: multiple sclerosis treatment; escalating strategy; he-DMT; diseases modifying therapies; early intense therapy

1. Introduction

1.1. Multiple Sclerosis: A General Overview

Multiple sclerosis (MS) is a disorder of remarkable heterogeneity that affects the central nervous system. It is characterized by inflammatory attacks to the myelin and axons, and by neurodegenerative cascade that give rise to progression of the disease independent of the initial inflammatory activity [1,2].

Based on these immunopathogenic mechanisms we can find two clinical forms of onset: bout-onset and progressive-onset disease. Bout-onset multiple sclerosis (BOMS) is characterized by relapses and remission (hence, relapsing-remitting MS (RRMS)). More than 50% of patients with BOMS will develop after variable time sustained progression of disability independent of the relapses, and hence, will convert to secondary progressive MS (SPMS). On the other hand, progressive-onset MS (POMS), is characterized by a sustained worsening of the disability since the beginning of the disease (hence, primary progressive MS [PPMS]) [3,4].

Relapses and progression are the main determinants of disability in MS [5]. However, natural history studies show that once progression becomes clinically evident, disability is no longer determined by the presence of previous relapses, and therefore is independent of the clinical form of onset (either BOMS or POMS). In fact, relapses have been shown to be minor contributors of progression of the disease. Specifically, short time between the first and second relapse and a sudden increase in the relapse rate in the preceding two years

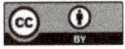

have been linked to the risk of developing SPMS, and yet they have little or no impact on disability once the progression has started [6,7].

At this point, two concepts must be introduced: relapse-associated worsening (RAW); the determinant of disability in RRMS, and steady progression independent of relapse activity (PIRA); the main determinant of disability in SPMS and PPMS [8–10]. Two other important considerations must be considered: the uncertainty of the real disease onset, and the lifelong duration of the disease. The diagnosis of MS is made based on the presence of relapses or sustained progression of disability in conjunction with typical magnetic resonance imaging and/or cerebrospinal fluid features. Therefore, it is important to recognize that the diagnosis may not truly mark the real onset of the disease, but rather the time at which the disease becomes clinically apparent and fulfills our established criteria to minimize the risk of misdiagnosis. Furthermore, BOMS is diagnosed around thirty years old, and SPMS and PPMS around forty-five years old. Considering life expectancy may be reduced by 5–7 years on average, it means that the average disease duration will be of 50 years for BOPMS and 35 years for POMS. These facts must be considered when analyzing clinical trials, as the apparent clinical disease duration may not be representative of the real disease duration, (thereby acting as a confounding factor), and because the follow-up times of these trials are too short to evaluate the impact over the long-term of the disease [11].

Continuing with the uncertainty surrounding MS, one of the main problems we face in treating MS is whether there is activation of the innate immune system, which has been linked to the progression of disability, from the onset of the disease or whether it occurs at some point as a result of dysregulation of the acquired immune system joint to the phenomenon of antigenic spread. There is currently no answer to this question, but very early initiation with induction drugs that reset the immune system, such as Alemtuzumab, have given the best results in terms of long-term progressive secondary progressive progression, which may indicate that intense early treatment could prevents activation of the innate immune system and triggering of the innate immune-dependent mechanisms responsible for the progression of the disability.

1.2. The Selection of the Objective in Clinical Trials

According to natural history studies and previous knowledge of the disease, the two main clinical endpoints chosen in phase III trials have been relapses and progression of disability [12]. When correlation between relapses and gadolinium-enhancing lesions (GEL) in the MRI was proven, it was also introduced as a surrogate marker of disease activity in phase II trials [13–16]. In fact, phase II trials have now replaced annualized relapses rate (ARR) with number of GEL as the primary endpoint, becoming the former a secondary endpoint, which has allowed trials to be shortened to six months. Meanwhile, phase III trials have maintained clinically defined primary endpoints: ARR for RRMS trials, and time to sustained progression confirmed in 3 or 6 months for PPMS trials [17].

Clinical secondary objectives in RRMS have been time to sustained progression of disability confirmed at 3 or 6 months. With the introduction of the MRI, T2 lesion number and volume, GEL number, and more recently, brain atrophy measures have been implemented in clinical trials [18]. However, it is important to consider the limited effect that these primary endpoints have in the natural history of the disease (i.e., development progressive course) and the potential confounding between relapse-related worsening and progressive disease [11]. This may explain the discrepancy observed between short-term efficacy of DMT on EDSS (mostly dependent on disability accumulation due to relapses) and the absence of effect to delay conversion to SPMS and to slow down progression of disability in PPMS and SPMS. An approach to deal with this problem has been to introduce the aforementioned concept of PIRA in clinical trials, as a way to distinguish progression of disability independent of relapses [19].

Also, scales other than EDSS such as the Multiple Sclerosis Functional Composite (MSFC), and other clinical and radiological variables, have been introduced to increase the sensitivity of progression of disability. However, uncertainty regarding the real clinical impact of these measures has limited their use [20,21].

Finally, care must be taken when assessing the clinical endpoint of a clinical trial. Firstly, the ARR may not harvest all the "focal" inflammatory activity. Secondly, ordinary brain MRI monitoring may fail to detect cortical lesions and ectopic meningeal follicles. Thirdly, progression measured by the EDSS is insensitive to minor clinical changes, especially when related to cognition [2].

For these reasons, treatment strategy in MS must be based on a judicious interpretation of the evidence from clinical trials. Special attention should be given to the actual results observed, as they may not reflect the reality of the disease and long-term effectiveness.

1.3. Classification of Disease Modifying Therapies

Before 1993, MS treatment was based on several immunosuppressive drugs, but it was with the approval of interferon (IFN) beta-1b (Betaferon®) that a new era of MS treatment began. Since then, nineteen drugs have been approved and four are already in the process of approval by the regulatory agencies. Obviously, each drug has a particular mechanism of action (MoA), level of effectiveness, and safety profile. According to the decrease in the ARR, DMT have been classified as moderate-intermediate efficacy and high-efficacy therapies (HET). IFN, glatiramer acetate (GA), azathioprine, and the newer orals drugs teriflunomide and dimethyl fumarte (dimethyl fumarate) are usually considered as being of moderate efficacy. Fingolimod, other sphingosine-1-phosphate (S1P) receptor modulators and cladribine are usually considered as intermediate efficacy drugs. Finally, monoclonal antibodies (MoAb) such natalizumab, alemtuzumab and ocrelizumab, together with mitoxantrone (an antineoplastic agent) are usually considered HET. Daclizumab, a MoAb, is no longer considered as a treatment for MS due to severe and unacceptable secondary effects [22–34].

Aside to this classification, DMT have been also classified as "first-line" therapies and "second-line" therapies. The former, DMTs of moderate efficacy but low side effects profile such IFN, GA, teriflunomide and dimethyl fumarate are usually included. In the USA, fingolimod and cladribine are also considered as "first-line" DMT. "Second-line" therapies include the MoAb and mitoxantrone. The use of these terms is applicable for the treatment of RRMS, but not for PPMS and SPMS [35].

Classification of DMT into "lines" of treatment has been the most popular one, and this has determined the escalation-based treatment approach, despite the absence of clinical evidence and disparities in this classification. For example, fingolimod is considered as a "second-line" drug in Europe, but a first-line drug in the USA. On the other hand, dimethyl fumarate, despite having several cases of progressive multifocal leukoencephalopathy (PML), is considered a first-line therapy. Additionally, cladribine, which is approved in Europe for highly active RRMS, and in the USA also for relapsing forms SPMS, has not been robustly studied in either of these settings.

For more than 25 years, this absurd classification into lines of treatment that implies an escalation approach strategy has prevailed. The question arises as to whether this is the best approach when considering the long-term impact on the disease [36].

1.4. The Concept of Treatment Failure

The first double blind randomized placebo controlled clinical trial in RRMS, tested IFN-1b against placebo. After three years, the number of relapse-free patients was 17/123 (13.8%) in the placebo arm; and 27/124 (21.7%) in the treated-arm [37]. It was clear that almost 2/3 of patients had relapses despite treatment. Consequently, three lines of investigation were established: to identify non-responders; to define baseline characteristics of non-responders; and to study the consequences of a suboptimal response. All these lines of investigations prompted a definition of treatment failure (TF) or suboptimal response (RSO). Waubant et al. were the first authors to define TF, based on the relapse rate, and defining TF as an ARR similar to the previous year [38]. Rio et al. used different criteria to define TF, as it included progression of EDSS, and a combination of clinical activity and MRI outcomes. However, progression of EDSS was a confounding factor, as IFN was not intended to treat progression. Sormani then modified these criteria (hence, the modified Rio-Sormani score), which remain as the most widely accepted definition of TF in current studies [39,40].

It is important to highlight that that the modified Rio-Sormani score has only been validated with IFN-1b treatment. If we want to apply these criteria in current clinical practice, we must consider the real value of a drug and the consequences of TF. For example, if a given drug is not intended to treat progression, it is reasonable that TF should not be considered when treatment has no effect on progression.

In agreement with this idea, it does not seem reasonable to consider TF when a progressive increases in disability are demonstrated under a determinate treatment, if the treatment have no effect over progression, at the same time, the presence of some inflammatory activity in form of relapses and/or MRI activity, are expected.

The short duration of clinical trials and observational studies has set the focus on the short-term effect of DMTs over disability, leading to the escalation strategy. However, long-term studies show DMT have a scarce effect on the risk of conversion to the SPMS and on disability once the progressive phase has started. This raises the question as to whether an escalation approach therapy is really appropriate [9,41].

Furthermore, if we follow the principle primum non nocere ("first, do no harm"), we should be cautious when escalating therapy, as HET initiation years after the disease increase the likelihood adverse events, but still do not change the long-term prognosis of the disease. HET have shown to have a greatest effect on the risk of conversion to SPMS when initiated early in the disease, during the so-called "window of opportunity". Still, early treatment with HET may expose young, healthy individuals with minor disability to serious side effects. Thus, the real debate should be whether the risks of early initiation HET outweigh the risks over the long term, and not where early intense therapy is "more efficacious" than escalation therapy.

2. Escalation Therapy

2.1. Definition

Escalation therapy must be clearly defined to compare studies and management strategies consistently. A European survey about MS management showed that treatment escalation or initiation based on relapses or new T2 lesions varied significantly between different countries, territories and even at institutions themselves [42]. There was a high agreement in switching to a HET when a patient experienced either two relapses, 5–8 new T2 lesions or two gadolinium enhancing lesions within a year [43]. However, this threshold is probably too high since these patients have a high probability to develop SPMS in the next two years. Hence, to evaluate the impact of treatment escalation, studies must clearly define previous DMTs, time evolution of the disease, and most importantly, the reason for treatment escalation. Otherwise, these studies may lead to paradoxical results, as was the case in the based on one of the largest registries of patients with multiple sclerosis, the MSBase registry, which used propensity score methodology, showed that patients starting on HET (fingolimod, alemtuzumab or natalizumab) had lower probability of conversion to SPMS when compared to patients starting on GA or IFN. In this series, time to treatment initiation was 6.5 years for HET vs. 5.1 years for GA or IFN. Furthermore, the authors reported a lower risk of conversion to SPMS when GA or IFN was started within 5 years versus later. In fact, treatment escalation after 5 years of evolution did not have a clear effect on the probability of converting to SPMS [43].

These evidence highlights the importance in defining to whom and to what DMT is being changed, as this is they are the only way to obtain clear conclusions from the escalation-based treatment strategy. It is not an academic question, as data shows that timing of treatment is crucial to impact significantly the probability to convert to SPMS, which might be related to effects of an aging immune system (i.e., immunosenescence) and loss of a potential "window of opportunity", which evidence suggests is limited to around 5 years.

2.2. Trials That Support Escalation Therapy

The currently approved HET are: natalizumab, fingolimod, alemtuzumab, ocrelizumab and cladribine. However, only fingolimod, alemtuzumab and ocrelizumab have been studied in appropriate clinical trials and have class A evidence of superiority with respect to other first-line therapies.

2.2.1. Fingolimod

The TRANSFORMS trial, fingolimod was assessed against IFN beta 1-a for one year in patients with RRMS between 18 and 55 years [44]. Patients had to have a relapse within the previous year, or two relapses within the previous two years, and a EDSS score between 0 and 5.5. 1292 patients were randomized: 426 to fingolimod 1.25 mg once a day; 431 to fingolimod 0.5 mg once a day-; and 435 to follow with IFN beta 1-a 30 µg i.m. weekly. The main clinical results were a reduction of the ARR of 0.16 in the 0.5 mg fingolimod arm, vs. 0.33 in the IFN beta 1-a arm; 82.6% of relapse-free patients in the 0.5 mg fingolimod arm vs. 69.3% in the IFN beta-1-a arm; and no differences with respect to progression of disability after one year. The main criticism of this trial (and other subsequent trials) is that the "active" treatment was continued even during a suboptimal response. Moreover, 45% of patients already had been treated with a previous DMT. Therefore, is difficult to draw conclusions about the effect of a treatment when is compared to another that has previously failed in these patients. Even so, the main clinical endpoint (progression of disability) was not met. Moreover, the extension trial at two years, despite having good results in MRI variables, still did not show any significant differences in progression of disability.

2.2.2. Alemtuzumab

The second HET that was explored against an active comparator in naïve patients or that failed to a previous treatment was alemtuzumab. This was assessed in the two-phase III clinical trials: the CARE-MS I and the CARE-MS II. In the former, 581 naïve patients with RRMS were randomized in a 2:1 proportion to receive either alemtuzumab 12 mg or Rebif-44 3 days a week and followed up for two years. The main results were a reduction of the ARR of 0.18 in the alemtuzumab arm vs. 0.39 in the Rebif-44 arm, and 77.6% of relapses-free patients in the alemtuzumab arm vs. 58.7% in the Rebif-44 arm. There were no differences in sustained accumulation of disability confirmed over 6 months between groups, possibly due to the low baseline disability of patients. In the CARE-MS II trial, 636 RRMS patients with at least one relapse while on GA or IFN beta were randomized in 2:1 proportion to receive alemtuzumab 12 mg or Rebif-44. After two years, 65.4% in the alemtuzumab 12 mg arm remained relapse-free vs. 46.7% in the Tebif-44 arm. Unlike CARE-MS I, this trial showed a lower rate of sustained confirmed progression at 6 months in the alemtuzumab arm (13% vs. 20%). There was also a positive effect over the MSFC score and MRI measures. Hence, CARE-MS II, which used a population with higher inflammatory activity (previous treatment failure) and higher EDSS, did show a clear effect on disability accumulation [45,46].

2.2.3. Ocrelizumab

The development phase III program of ocrelizumab in RRMS was done in two simultaneous and identical trials: OPERA-I and OPERA-II. Inclusion criteria required at least one relapse within the previous 2 years. These trials randomized a total of 1656 patients in a 1:1 ratio to receive ocrelizumab or Rebif-44. 71% and 73% were treatment naïve. The main results in the pooled analyses were a reduction in the ARR (0.16 in the ocrelizumab arm vs. 0.29 in the Rebif-44 arm), and a reduction in the proportion of patients reaching disability progression confirmed at 12 weeks (9.1% vs. 13.6%, respectively). However, subgroup analyses suggested that the reduction of progression of disability was not significant among the 224 patients that were previously treated with a DMT, despite having a positive effect on the ARR. Similarly, subgroup analyses showed that the reduction of progression was not significant when considering patients with a body mass index of 25 or more. This example of "tortured-data", seems to suggest ocrelizumab may be more effective in lean than overweight patients [47,48].

2.3. Summary

The efficacy of escalation to HET has been evaluated in a myriad of observational studies, but level A evidence supporting this strategy is scarce. Although evidence shows that escalation therapy is useful to abrogate inflammatory activity, it has only showed a modest effect over the progression of disability. In fact, the longest observational studies still show that this strategy is futile to prevent conversion to SPMS. However, this does not prove that this strategy is not valid. We might consider it as a useful therapy to reduce relapses and the progression of disability in the beginning of the disease. Data suggest that beyond four or five years, the effect on relapses maintains, but not on accumulation of disability.

3. High-Efficacy Therapy

3.1. Definition

High-efficacy therapy (HET) refers to agents that have a greater impact on inflammation compared to moderately effective therapies [49]. Therefore, the classification of DMT as high-efficacy is based on favorable outcomes from clinical trials comparing that treatment usually to traditional DMTs (mostly inflammatory outcomes such as relapses and new lesions, although some experts prefer to evaluate lack of disability too) [49].

There is an agreement to consider natalizumab, antiCD20 therapy (rituximab and ocrelizumab), alemtuzumab, mitoxantrone, cyclophosphamide and autologous stem cell transplantation as HET. However, there is not a consensus regarding sphingosine-1-phosphate receptor modulators such as fingolimod (some consider it an intermediate efficacy therapy) and cladribine (as it has been compared to placebo, although it probably has an induction effect) [49] (Table 1).

Table 1. Early Intensive Therapy. * There is not consensus regarding Cladribine and fingolimod (as some authors consider them HET and others not).

Early Intensive Therapy (EIT):	
Induction Treatment	Mitoxantrone Cyclophosphamide Stem Cell transplantation Alemtuzumab Cladribine *
Sustained High-Efficacy Treatment	Natalizumab Fingolimod * Anti-CD20 treatment

As opposed to escalation, where treatment starts with a low-risk and lower-efficacy treatment and only moves on to a more aggressive treatment if the ongoing approach fails, early aggressive therapy or Early Intensive Therapy (EIT) considers starting high-efficacy treatment earlier in MS, mostly initially since its onset, to maximize the potential for preventing disability progression over time, assuming a higher-risk profile of adverse events [48,50].

Many consider that EIT as the best way to achieve long-term outcomes for people with MS, based on the following rationale: the ability to predict disease course at onset is limited, conventional imaging underestimates ongoing damage, irreversible nervous damage occurs very early and once neurological function is lost it cannot be regained. MS is rarely benign over the long term. Long term follow-up studies reveal the risks of undertreatment. Safety profile of some HET may not differ from low-efficacy treatment and it is mainly early intervention that might substantively alter disease course and prevent irreversible progression, whereas later treatment might not confer much benefit [3–9]. Therefore, EIT is based on using highly effective treatments starting early, while on the therapeutic window, where they are more effective than when started later on the disease course in the escalation approach [51–57] (Table 2).

Table 2. Long-term outcomes of Early Intensive Treatments: Observational Studies.

Beneficial Long-Term Outcomes of EIT vs. Escalation		
Observational Studies	Follow-Up	Outcomes
Buron et al. [58]	4 years	Lower risk of 6 month EDSS worsening and of first relapse
Harding et al. [59]	5 years	Lower increase in EDSS Longer Median time to sustained accumulation of disability
He et al. [60]	6–10 years	Early HET within 2 years of disease onset is associated with lower hazard of disability progression and lower disability accumulation at 6 to 10 years of follow-up compared to late HET
Iaffaldano et al. [61]	10 years	Lower disability progression measured by mean annual EDSS change compared to baseline value in all time points, including at 5 and 10 years.
Brown et al. [46]	5.8 years	Lower risk of conversion to SPMS
Prosperini et al. [62]	10 years	Lower proportion of patients reached the milestone of EDSS 6 at 10 years

However, when considering EIT, two main approaches arise. Firstly, Induction treatment (IT), also referred to as immune reconstitution therapy which is based on the use of HET with a sustained biological effect in naïve patients, followed or not by long-term maintenance treatment (generally with immunomodulatory agents) and secondly, sustained HET, which is based on the use of HET continuously, as their effect wanes when interrupting treatment [50–57]. Induction treatment includes mitoxantrone, cyclophosphamide, stem cell transplantation, alemtuzumab and cladribine, whereas the potential inductive effect of antiCD20 therapy is mild and of natalizumab and fingolimod is null (as their withdrawal is associated with reactivation of the disease) [50–56]. Induction treatments usually are associated with a higher risk profile but shorter in time as their administration is not sustained, while the use of continuous HET is associated with a risk profile sustained overtime. The rationale for induction therapy is to influence the inflammatory phase and to avoid the subsequent chronic phase resetting the immunological system to prevent the phenomenon of epitope spread [50–52]. The risk associated with treatment that is judged acceptable may vary with disease severity, however, disease severity might be underestimated, specially early at onset, and treatments are less effective as disease evolves [51,54–56]. It is known that MS patients treated early do better than those in whom treatment is delayed, but regarding the question does the potency of DMT truly matter, recent observational studies show better long-term outcomes on disability accumulation and risk of conversion to SPMS with EIT than escalation [57].

3.2. Results over Inflammatory Activity, Progression, and Safety

Natalizumab's original trial, AFFIRM study, showed a 68% reduction in ARR at year 1, 42% relative risk reduction in disability progression at 2 years, 83% reduction of new T2 lesions and 92% reduction in contrast enhancing lesions compared to placebo. The REVEAL study compared natalizumab to fingolimod with a lower cumulative probability of relapse and gadolinium-enhancing lesions 70% lower in the natalizumab group. Several observational studies comparing naive patients treated with natalizumab vs. injectables DMT have shown greater reductions in ARR and disability accrual, and others, when comparing escalation to Natalizumab to those switching to fingolimod have shown higher rates of NEDA with natalizumab. The TOP study at 5 years reported lower ARR in naive natalizumab patients than those who escalated to natalizumab from prior DMTs. Natalizumab main risk are infusion related reactions and PML risk [49,63].

Regarding Alemtuzumab, phase II CAMMS223 in naive RRMS showed better results on relapses, disability accumulation, MRI activity and atrophy compared to interferon at 3 years. In the CARE-MS I study with naive RRMS alemtuzumab reduced significantly ARR and MRI activity at 2 years but not disability progression compared to interferon-beta-1A, and in the CARE-MS 2 study with RRMS who failed to previous DMT, alemtuzumab reduced the ARR, MRI and disability progression at 2 years compared to interferon. Extension studies up to 6 years showed sustained benefits of alemtuzumab on clinical and MRI activity and progression of disability in a great proportion of patients, and interestingly the conversion rate to SPMS at 6 years was very low (3%). A cohort study comparing alemtuzumab effectiveness to natalizumab, fingolimod and interferons, up to 5 years, revealed similar reductions on ARR for alemtuzumab and natalizumab, but superior to fingolimod and interferons, however natalizumab seemed better than alemtuzumab in enabling recovery from disability. Alemtuzumab safety risks include infusion reactions, stroke and arterial dissection, severe infections including opportunistic ones such as herpetic and Listeria monocytogenes, and secondary autoimmune disorders (thyroid disorders, idiopathic thrombocytopenic purpura, and nephropathies among others) [49,50,63–66].

Cladribine was studied in the 2-year placebo-controlled phase 3 study CLARITY, with lower relapse rates, lower risk of 3 months sustained disability progression and significant reductions in brain lesions counts. Moreover, the 2-year extension study of CLARITY showed that patients that received cladribine during the core study followed by placebo during the third and fourth year had sustained benefits in terms of activity and progression (similar to 4 years with cladribine treatment). However, Cladribine may be slightly less effective than other HET, as an observational study revealed a significant reduction on ARR with cladribine compared to medium efficacy therapies and a similar reduction compared to fingolimod, but a lower reduction compared to natalizumab. Cladribine safety issues are related mainly to lymphopenia and herpes zoster infections [49,50,64].

Rituximab is used off-label in MS. Rituximab compared to placebo in a phase II trial showed a lower risk of relapse and greater reductions on MRI activity. Several observational studies, especially from Sweden, have confirmed these results. Moreover, an observational study revealed that switching from natalizumab (due to JCV positivity) to rituximab was related to lower clinical and MRI activity compared to switching to fingolimod. In a comparative study with a 4-year follow-up, initial treatment with rituximab demonstrated a significant lower rate of relapses and MRI activity compared to injectable DMTs and dimethyl fumarate, with a tendency for lower relapse rates compared with natalizumab and fingolimod. The OPERA I and II phase III studies compared ocrelizumab to interferon-beta-1a in RRMS patients with greater reductions in ARR, MRI activity and progression of disability at 3 and 6 months with ocrelizumab. The most common side effects of anti-CD20 therapy are infusion reactions and infections (including cases of herpes zoster, hepatitis B reactivation and PML), although bone marrow suppression and neutropenia have been described [66,67].

Mitoxantrone was compared to placebo in a French-British randomized controlled trial and to Interferon-beta in a 3-year pivotal trial, and was related to a significant lower relapse rate, MRI activity and disability worsening. Another study compared induction with mitoxantrone followed by glatiramer acetate maintenance therapy vs. glatiramer acetate, with a significant reduction on ARR and MRI activity in the first group. Long-term mitoxantrone effectiveness has been studied up to 5–10 years of follow-up with significant results on reduction of disability worsening, compared to medium efficacy DMTs, especially when followed by platform treatment maintenance. The risk of severe adverse events such as heart failure or leukemia or amenorrhea make mitoxantrone a less suitable treatment option nowadays [49,50,62,64].

Regarding Cyclophosphamide, the two-year randomized clinical trial of cyclophosphamide followed by interferon vs. interferon alone showed a significant reduction in clinical and MRI activity, and an observational study using induction with cyclophosphamide followed by maintenance therapy with glatiramer acetate showed similar results. However, its safety profile mainly related to infections and hemorrhagic cystitis and bladder cancer have reduced its use nowadays [50,62].

Autologous hematopoietic stem cell transplantation (AHSCT) has been used in aggressive RRMS. The phase II ASTIMS trial demonstrated AHSCT was superior to mitoxantrone reducing relapse rates and MRI activity without differences in the progression of disability between groups. An observational study showed an important proportion of progression-free survival at 5 years of follow-up with AHSCT, with better outcomes with lower baseline EDSS. Another observational study revealed AHSCT is more suitable for aggressive RRMS as none of the RRMS experienced worsening of disability after a median follow-up of 5.4 years while 22.6% of SPMS experienced disability worsening. However, safety risks of AHSCT including infections and mortality, make AHSCT suitable only for aggressive RRMS patients refractory to high-efficacy conventional therapies and active disease with potential for disability accumulation. The BEAT-MS (Best Available Therapy Versus Autologous Hematopoietic Stem Cell Transplant for Multiple Sclerosis) study is a 6-year ongoing study currently investigating AHSCT versus high-efficacy DMTs (natalizumab, alemtuzumab, ocrelizumab, or rituximab) with a primary endpoint of relapse-free survival up to 36 months [49,50,68].

Interestingly, a recent Norwegian observational study has compared the short-term effect of initial HET (with natalizumab, fingolimod and alemtuzumab) vs. medium efficacy treatment. Initial HET was associated with a greater proportion of NEDA at years 1 and 2 compared to initial medium efficacy treatment (OR 3.9, $p < 0.001$, at year 1) [69].

3.3. The Importance of Long-Terms Outcomes. Analysis of the Comparative Studies: Escalation vs. Early Intensive Treatment

Initiating effective treatment early in the disease course in order to reduce relapse rate and the underlying inflammatory process may delay irreversible neurological damage and conversion to a secondary progressive course. The median time to conversion to a secondary progressive course is around fifteen years but can be shorter, especially in patients with aggressive disease [54]. The main goal of treatment must be to prevent accumulation of irreversible neurological disability and, in particular, to prevent conversion to a secondary progressive course [54].

However, clinical trials have short follow-up times, which might prevent detection of progression of disability and moreover disability worsening in these scenarios may reflect mainly disability accrual from relapses rather than true progression. Furthermore, extension phases have many biases that preclude long-term outcomes analysis, and moreover, clinical trials do not usually compare the escalation and EIT approach. Therefore, long-term outcomes that assess disability at five to ten years after treatment onset, and conversion to secondary progressive MS must be analyzed on real world experience.

Recent evidence from several observational studies, suggest that EIT provides a greater benefit than escalation treatment in decreasing the risk of developing SPMS and disability accrual at least in the medium-long term of 5 to 10 years [43,58–62].

A Danish observational study with 4 years follow-up showed that initial high efficacy treatment (with natalizumab, fingolimod, alemtuzumab, ocrelizumab or cladribine) compared to medium efficacy treatment in naive patients (using propensity score matched samples) was associated with a lower probability of 6-month confirmed EDSS worsening (16.7% vs. 30.1%, HR 0.53, $p = 0.006$) and of a first relapse (HR 0.50) up to 4 years. Although fingolimod was initially considered as HET, when reclassifying it as a medium DMT, comparable results as in the main study were found. When subgroup analysis of patients with high baseline disease activity was done, comparable results were found too [58].

Another real-life setting study showed long-term outcomes were more favorable following initial EIT (with natalizumab or alemtuzumab) vs. moderate-efficacy treatment (with interferons, glatiramer, teriflunomide, dimethyl fumarate and fingolimod). This cohort UK study that included 592 RRMS patients showed that EIT patients had a lower increase in EDSS score at 5 years than patients with the escalation approach (0.3 vs. 1.2, $p = 0.002$). Median time to sustained accumulation of disability was longer for the EIT, but no differences were found between the medium-efficacy DMT who escalated to high-efficacy DMT and the EIT group. However, 60% of those who escalated to HET had already developed disability accumulation while still receiving initial moderate-efficacy treatment before escalation. Despite this, patients that received initial EIT had a more active disease (pretreatment ARR 1.7 vs. 0.7), it was this group that had better long-term outcomes. Interestingly, age at onset of first DMT was also related to EDSS change at 5 years [59].

An observational study with data from the Swedish MS and MSBase registries, assessed the efficacy of HET (natalizumab, rituximab, ocrelizumab, alemtuzumab or mitoxantrone) started early (0–2 years from onset) compared to later (4–6 years from onset) using propensity score. Although this study did not compare efficacy with the escalation approach (and escalation was allowed in both groups), it proved that early HET within 2 years of disease onset is associated with lower hazard of disability progression and lower disability accumulation at 6 to 10 years of follow-up compared to late HET (mean EDSS score at 10 years: 2.3 vs. 3.5, $p < 0.0001$) [60].

An Italian multicentric study that analyzed long-term trajectories up to 10 years of EIT vs. escalation in naive RRMS, starting treatment within the first year of disease onset, demonstrated EIT strategy is more effective than escalation in controlling disability progression over time. In this study EIT included patients that received as first DMT fingolimod, natalizumab, mitoxantrone, alemtuzumab, ocrelizumab or cladribine while escalation group received the high efficacy DMT after at least 1 year of treatment with glatiramer acetate, interferons, azathioprine, teriflunomide or dimethyl fumarate. Patients were followed for 10 years, and propensity score matched for characteristics at first DMT before analysis, all having at least one relapse on the previous year and baseline mean EDSS of 2.6. EIT was significantly associated with lower disability progression measured by mean annual EDSS change compared to baseline value in all time points, including at 5 and 10 years. This effect not only persisted but continued to increase over time despite all patients in the escalation group being escalated to a higher-efficacy DMT [61].

Regarding conversion to SPMS, EIT has been associated with a lower risk of conversion than escalation. A multicentric cohort study with 1555 patients, using propensity score matching, showed that EIT (initial treatment with alemtuzumab, natalizumab and fingolimod) was associated with a lower risk of conversion to SPMS than initial treatment with interferons and glatiramer (HR 0.66, $p = 0.046$; with a 5-year absolute risk 7% vs. 12%, median follow-up, 5.8 years). However, the probability of conversion to SPMS was lower when interferons or glatiramer were started within 5 years of disease onset versus later, and when platform treatments were escalated to fingolimod, alemtuzumab or natalizumab within 5 years versus later (HR 0.76, $p < 0.001$, 5-year absolute risk 8% vs. 14%, median follow-up 5.3 years), which may reflect that when using the escalation approach, treatment failure must be promptly detected [43].

In relation to long-term outcomes of specifically induction treatment in observational studies, most of available data is mainly related to the older induction treatments such as mitoxantrone or cyclophosphamide compared to injectable medium-efficacy treatment. Prosperini et al., compared effects and safety of initial induction treatment with mitoxantrone or cyclophosphamide vs. escalation treatment starting with interferons in active RRMS (with median ARR of 2 and 60% of patients with baseline contrast enhancing lesions) using propensity score match, and found that a significantly lower proportion of patients of the induction group reached the milestone of EDSS 6 at 10 years (28% vs. 38.7%, HR

0.48, $p = 0.024$). Younger age was related with better outcomes in the induction group, and adverse events were more frequent after induction. Notably, although induction was not compared with initial sustained HET, some of the induction patients required escalation to fingolimod or other monoclonal antibodies, however, in a lower proportion than the escalation group (34.7% vs. 53.4%) [62].

Data related to newer induction treatments such as alemtuzumab or cladribine are usually analyzed together with other HET versus the escalation approach, but no observational studies of long-term outcomes comparing initial induction versus initial sustained HET are available [62].

Therefore, real-world data show that the escalation approach may be inadequate to prevent long-term outcomes compared to EIT and that initial EIT is related to a lower risk of developing SPMS and to lower disability accumulation at 5 and 10 years. However, evidence comparing long-term outcomes of induction treatment vs. sustained HET is scarce [58–60,62].

4. Future Evidence

To assess the effectiveness of EIT vs. Escalation, two pivotal clinical trials are currently ongoing; the TREAT-MS (TRaditional versus Early Aggressive Therapy for MS) trial and the DELIVER-MS (Determining the Effectiveness of earLy Intensive Versus Escalation approaches for the treatment of Relapsing-remitting MS) trial. The primary endpoint in TREAT-MS is time to sustained disability progression and the primary endpoint in DELIVER-MS is normalized whole brain volume loss from baseline to month 36. Interestingly both clinical trials consider the sphingosine-1-P modulators as medium efficacy treatments, while the first one considers cladribine as an EIT and the last one as a medium efficacy treatment [49,61,62].

This work has been supported by a grant from the Health Institute Carlos III: PI20/01446.

Authors should discuss the results and how they can be interpreted from the perspective of previous studies and of the working hypotheses. The findings and their implications should be discussed in the broadest context possible. Future research directions may also be highlighted.

Author Contributions: Conceptualization, B.C. and F.G.; methodology, B.C., C.Q.-B. and F.G.; formal analysis, B.C.; investigation, B.C. and F.G.; writing—original draft preparation, B.C., C.Q.-B. and F.G.; writing—review and editing, C.Q.-B.; supervision, B.C. All authors have read and agreed to the published version of the manuscript.

Funding: This research was funded by a grant from the Health Institute Carlos III: PI20/01446.

Conflicts of Interest: The authors declare no conflict of interest.

References

1. Lassmann, H.; Brück, W.; Lucchinetti, C.F. The Immunopathology of Multiple Sclerosis: An Overview. *Brain Pathol.* **2007**, *17*, 210–218. [CrossRef]
2. Frischer, J.M.; Bramow, S.; Dal-Bianco, A.; Lucchinetti, C.F.; Rauschka, H.; Schmidbauer, M.; Laursen, H.; Sorensen, P.S.; Lassmann, H. The relation between inflammation and neurodegeneration in multiple sclerosis brains. *Brain* **2009**, *132*, 1175–1189. [CrossRef] [PubMed]
3. Lublin, F.D.; Reingold, S.C.; Cohen, J.A.; Cutter, G.R.; Sørensen, P.S.; Thompson, A.J.; Wolinsky, J.S.; Balcer, L.J.; Banwell, B.; Barkhof, F.; et al. Defining the clinical course of multiple sclerosis: The 2013 revisions. *Neurology* **2014**, *83*, 278–286. [CrossRef]
4. Tutuncu, M.; Tang, J.; Zeid, N.A.; Kale, N.; Crusan, D.J.; Atkinson, E.J.; Siva, A.; Pittock, S.J.; Pirko, I.; Keegan, B.M.; et al. Onset of progressive phase is an age-dependent clinical milestone in multiple sclerosis. *Mult. Scler. J.* **2013**, *19*, 188–198. [CrossRef]
5. Tremlett, H.; Zhao, Y.; Rieckmann, P.; Hutchinson, M. New perspectives in the natural history of multiple sclerosis. *Neurology* **2010**, *74*, 2004–2015. [CrossRef] [PubMed]
6. Confavreux, C.; Vukusic, S.; Moreau, T.; Adeleine, P. Relapses and progression of disability in Multiple Sclerosis. *N. Engl. J. Med.* **2000**, *343*, 1430–1438. [CrossRef] [PubMed]
7. Shirani, A.; Okuda, D.; Stüve, O. Therapeutic Advances and Future Prospects in Progressive Forms of Multiple Sclerosis. *Neurotherapeutics* **2016**, *13*, 58–69. [CrossRef]

8. Novotna, M.; Soldán, M.M.P.; Zeid, N.A.; Kale, N.; Tutuncu, M.; Crusan, D.J.; Atkinson, E.J.; Siva, A.; Keegan, B.M.; Pirko, I.; et al. Poor early relapse recovery affects onset of progressive disease course in multiple sclerosis. *Neurology* **2015**, *85*, 722–729. [CrossRef]
9. Cree, B.A.C.; Gourraud, P.-A.; Oksenberg, J.R.; Bevan, C.; Crabtree-Hartman, E.; Gelfand, J.M.; Goodin, D.S.; Graves, J.; Green, A.J.; Mowry, E.; et al. Long-term evolution of multiple sclerosis disability in the treatment era. *Ann. Neurol.* **2016**, *80*, 499–510. [CrossRef]
10. Cree, B.A.C.; Hollenbach, J.A.; Bove, R.; Kirkish, G.; Sacco, S.; Caverzasi, E.; Bischof, A.; Gundel, T.; Zhu, A.H.; Papinutto, N.; et al. Silent progression in disease activity–free relapsing multiple sclerosis. *Ann. Neurol.* **2019**, *85*, 653–666. [CrossRef]
11. Scalfari, A.; Neuhaus, A.; Daumer, M.; Muraro, P.A.; Ebers, G.C. Onset of secondary progressive phase and long-term evolution of multiple sclerosis. *J. Neurol. Neurosurg. Psychiatr.* **2014**, *85*, 67–75. [CrossRef] [PubMed]
12. Ebers, G.C.; Heigenhauser, L.; Daumer, M.; Lederer, C.; Noseworthy, J.H. Disability as an outcome in MS clinical trials. *Neurology* **2008**, *71*, 624–631. [CrossRef]
13. Silver, N.; Good, C.; Sormani, M.; MacManus, D.; Thompson, A.; Filippi, M.; Miller, D. A modified protocol to improve the detection of enhancing brain and spinal cord lesions in multiple sclerosis. *J. Neurol.* **2001**, *248*, 215–224. [CrossRef]
14. Signori, A.; Gallo, F.; Bovis, F.; Di Tullio, N.; Maietta, I.; Sormani, M.P. Long-term impact of interferon or Glatiramer acetate in multiple sclerosis: A systematic review and meta-analysis. *Mult. Scler. Relat. Disord.* **2016**, *6*, 57–63. [CrossRef]
15. Sormani, M.P.; Rovaris, M.; Comi, G.; Filippi, M. A composite score to predict short-term disease activity in patients with relapsing-remitting MS. *Neurology* **2007**, *69*, 1230–1235. [CrossRef] [PubMed]
16. Sormani, M.P.; de Stefano, N. Defining and scoring response to IFN-β in multiple sclerosis. *Nat. Rev. Neurol.* **2013**, *9*, 504–512. [CrossRef] [PubMed]
17. Gehr, S.; Kaiser, T.; Kreutz, R.; Ludwig, W.-D.; Paul, F. Suggestions for improving the design of clinical trials in multiple sclerosis—Results of a systematic analysis of completed phase III trials. *EPMA J.* **2019**, *10*, 425–436. [CrossRef]
18. de Stefano, N.; Giorgio, A.; Battaglini, M.; Rovaris, M.; Sormani, M.P.; Barkhof, F.; Korteweg, T.; Enzinger, C.; Fazekas, F.; Calabrese, M.; et al. Assessing brain atrophy rates in a large population of untreated multiple sclerosis subtypes. *Neurology* **2010**, *74*, 1868–1876. [CrossRef]
19. Kappos, L.; Wolinsky, J.S.; Giovannoni, G.; Arnold, D.L.; Wang, Q.; Bernasconi, C.; Model, F.; Koendgen, H.; Manfrini, M.; Belachew, S.; et al. Contribution of Relapse-Independent Progression vs Relapse-Associated Worsening to Overall Confirmed Disability Accumulation in Typical Relapsing Multiple Sclerosis in a Pooled Analysis of 2 Randomized Clinical Trials. *JAMA Neurol.* **2020**, *77*, 1132–1140. [CrossRef]
20. Rotstein, D.L.; Healy, B.C.; Malik, M.T.; Chitnis, T.; Weiner, H.L. Evaluation of No Evidence of Disease Activity in a 7-Year Longitudinal Multiple Sclerosis Cohort. *JAMA Neurol.* **2015**, *72*, 152–158. [CrossRef]
21. Mahajan, K.R.; Ontaneda, D. The Role of Advanced Magnetic Resonance Imaging Techniques in Multiple Sclerosis Clinical Trials. *Neurotherapeutics* **2017**, *14*, 905–923. [CrossRef]
22. Kappos, L.; Freedman, M.S.; Polman, C.H.; Edan, G.; Hartung, H.-P.; Miller, D.H.; Montalban, X.; Barkhof, F.; Radü, E.-W.; Metzig, C.; et al. Long-term effect of early treatment with interferon beta-1b after a first clinical event suggestive of multiple sclerosis: 5-year active treatment extension of the phase 3 BENEFIT trial. *Lancet Neurol.* **2009**, *8*, 987–997. [CrossRef]
23. Johnson, K.P.; Brooks, B.R.; Cohen, J.A.; Ford, C.C.; Goldstein, J.; Lisak, R.P.; Myers, L.W.; Panitch, H.S.; Rose, J.W.; Schiffer, R.B.; et al. Copolymer 1 reduces relapse rate and improves disability in relapsing-remitting multiple sclerosis: Results of a phase III multicenter, double-blind, placebo-controlled trial. *Neurology* **1995**, *45*, 1268–1276. [CrossRef] [PubMed]
24. Avasarala, J. Anti-CD20 Cell Therapies in Multiple Sclerosis—A Fixed Dosing Schedule for Ocrelizumab is Overkill. *Drug Target Insights* **2017**, *11*, 10–12. [CrossRef] [PubMed]
25. Kilpatrick, T.J.; Butzkueven, H. Immunosuppressive therapy is valuable in aggressive Multiple Sclerosis. *J. Clin. Neurosci.* **2000**, *7*, 561–563. [CrossRef]
26. Perumal, J.; Reardon, J. Review of daclizumab and its therapeutic potential in the treatment of relapsing–remitting multiple sclerosis. *Drug Des. Dev. Ther.* **2013**, *7*, 1187–1193. [CrossRef] [PubMed]
27. McCune, W.J.; Gonzalez-Rivera, T. Immunosuppressive Drug Therapy. *Dubois' Lupus Erythematosus Relat. Syndr.* **2013**, *2012*, 609–625. [CrossRef]
28. Byrne, E.; Panitch, H.; Coyle, P.; Goodin, D.; O'Connor, P.; Weinshenker, B.; Li, D.; Francis, G.; Chang, P.; Monaghan, E.; et al. Randomized, comparative study of interferon beta-1a treatment regimens in MS: The EVIDENCE trial. *Neurology* **2003**, *60*, 1872–1873. [CrossRef]
29. O'Connor, P.; Comi, G.; Freedman, M.S.; Miller, A.E.; Kappos, L.; Bouchard, J.-P.; Lebrun-Frenay, C.; Mares, J.; Benamor, M.; Thangavelu, K.; et al. Long-term safety and efficacy of teriflunomide. *Neurology* **2016**, *86*, 920–930. [CrossRef]
30. Gold, R.; Kappos, L.; Arnold, D.L.; Bar-Or, A.; Giovannoni, G.; Selmaj, K.; Tornatore, C.; Sweetser, M.T.; Yang, M.S.M.; Sheikh, S.I.; et al. Placebo-Controlled Phase 3 Study of Oral BG-12 for Relapsing Multiple Sclerosis. *N. Engl. J. Med.* **2012**, *367*, 1098–1107. [CrossRef]
31. Kappos, L.; O'Connor, P.; Radue, E.-W.; Polman, C.; Hohlfeld, R.; Selmaj, K.; Ritter, S.; Schlosshauer, R.; Von Rosenstiel, P.; Zhang-Auberson, L.; et al. Long-term effects of fingolimod in multiple sclerosis: The randomized FREEDOMS extension trial. *Neurology* **2015**, *84*, 1582–1591. [CrossRef] [PubMed]

32. Comi, G.; Cook, S.D.; Giovannoni, G.; Rammohan, K.; Rieckmann, P.; Sorensen, P.S.; Vermersch, P.; Hamlett, A.C.; Viglietta, V.; Greenberg, S.J. MRI outcomes with cladribine tablets for multiple sclerosis in the CLARITY study. *J. Neurol.* **2013**, *260*, 1136–1146. [CrossRef]
33. Freedman, M.S. Treatment options for patients with multiple sclerosis who have a suboptimal response to interferon-β therapy. *Eur. J. Neurol.* **2013**, *21*, 377-e20. [CrossRef]
34. Coles, A.J.; Twyman, C.L.; Arnold, D.L.; Cohen, J.A.; Confavreux, C.; Fox, E.J.; Hartung, H.-P.; Havrdova, E.K.; Selmaj, K.W.; Weiner, H.L.; et al. Alemtuzumab for patients with relapsing multiple sclerosis after disease-modifying therapy: A randomised controlled phase 3 trial. *Lancet* **2012**, *380*, 1829–1839. [CrossRef]
35. Gajofatto, A.; Benedetti, M.D. Treatment strategies for multiple sclerosis: When to start, when to change, when to stop? *World J. Clin. Cases* **2015**, *3*, 545–555. [CrossRef] [PubMed]
36. Huygens, S.; Versteegh, M. Modeling the Cost-Utility of Treatment Sequences for Multiple Sclerosis. *Value Health* **2021**, *24*, 1612–1619. [CrossRef] [PubMed]
37. O'Rourke, K.E.T.; Hutchinson, M. Stopping beta-interferon therapy in multiple sclerosis: An analysis of stopping patterns. *Mult. Scler. J.* **2005**, *11*, 46–50. [CrossRef]
38. Waubant, E.; Vukusic, S.; Gignoux, L.; Durand-Dubief, F.; Achiti, I.; Blanc, S.; Renoux, C.; Confavreux, C. Clinical characteristics of responders to interferon therapy for relapsing MS. *Neurology* **2003**, *61*, 184–189. [CrossRef]
39. Río, J.; Nos, C.; Tintore, M.; Borrás, C.; Galan, I.; Comabella, M.; Montalban, X. Assessment of different treatment failure criteria in a cohort of relapsing-remitting multiple sclerosis patients treated with interferon β: Implications for clinical trials. *Ann. Neurol.* **2002**, *52*, 400–406. [CrossRef]
40. Sormani, M.P.; Gasperini, C.; Romeo, M.; Rio, J.; Calabrese, M.; Cocco, E.; Enzingher, C.; Fazekas, F.; Filippi, M.; Gallo, A.; et al. Assessing response to interferon-β in a multicenter dataset of patients with MS. *Neurology* **2016**, *87*, 134–140. [CrossRef] [PubMed]
41. Gajofatto, A.; Bacchetti, P.; Grimes, B.; High, A.; Waubant, E. Switching first-line disease-modifying therapy after failure: Impact on the course of relapsing-remitting multiple sclerosis. *Mult. Scler. J.* **2009**, *15*, 50–58. [CrossRef] [PubMed]
42. Martinelli, V.; Comi, G. Induction versus escalation therapy. *Neurol. Sci.* **2005**, *26*, s193–s199. [CrossRef]
43. Brown, W.; Coles, A.; Horakova, D.; Havrdova, E.; Izquierdo, G.; Prat, A.; Girard, M.; Duquette, P.; Trojano, M.; Lugaresi, A.; et al. Association of Initial Disease-Modifying Therapy with Later Conversion to Secondary Progressive Multiple Sclerosis. *JAMA J. Am. Med. Assoc.* **2019**, *321*, 175–187. [CrossRef]
44. Fernández, O.; DelVecchio, M.; Edan, G.; Fredrikson, S.; Gionvannoni, G.; Hartung, H.-P.; Havrdova, E.K.; Kappos, L.; Pozzilli, C.; Soerensen, P.S.; et al. Survey of diagnostic and treatment practices for multiple sclerosis in Europe. *Eur. J. Neurol.* **2017**, *24*, 516–522. [CrossRef]
45. Cohen, J.A.; Barkhof, F.; Comi, G.; Hartung, H.-P.; Khatri, B.O.; Montalban, X.; Pelletier, J.; Capra, R.; Gallo, P.; Izquierdo, G.; et al. Oral Fingolimod or Intramuscular Interferon for Relapsing Multiple Sclerosis. *N. Engl. J. Med.* **2010**, *362*, 402–415. [CrossRef]
46. Cohen, J.A.; Coles, A.J.; Arnold, D.L.; Confavreux, C.; Fox, E.J.; Hartung, H.-P.; Havrdova, E.; Selmaj, K.W.; Weiner, H.L.; Fisher, E.; et al. Alemtuzumab versus interferon beta 1a as fi rst-line treatment for patients with relapsing-remitting multiple sclerosis: A randomised controlled phase 3 trial. *Lancet* **2012**, *380*, 1819–1828. [CrossRef]
47. Coles, A.J.; Cohen, J.A.; Fox, E.J.; Giovannoni, G.; Hartung, H.-P.; Havrdova, E.; Schippling, S.; Selmaj, K.W.; Traboulsee, A.; Compston, D.A.S. Alemtuzumab CARE-MS II 5-year Efficacy and safety findings. *Neurology* **2017**, *89*, 1117–1126. [CrossRef]
48. Hauser, S.L.; Bar-Or, A.; Comi, G.; Giovannoni, G.; Hartung, H.-P.; Hemmer, B.; Lublin, F.; Montalban, X.; Rammohan, K.W.; Selmaj, K.; et al. Ocrelizumab versus Interferon Beta-1a in Relapsing Multiple Sclerosis. *N. Engl. J. Med.* **2017**, *376*, 221–234. [CrossRef]
49. Simpson, A.; Mowry, E.M.; Newsome, S.D. Early Aggressive Treatment Approaches for Multiple Sclerosis. *Curr. Treat. Options Neurol.* **2021**, *23*, 1–21. [CrossRef] [PubMed]
50. Ruggieri, S.; Pontecorvo, S.; Tortorella, C.; Gasperini, C. Induction treatment strategy in multiple sclerosis: A review of past experiences and future perspectives. *Mult. Scler. Demyelinating Disord.* **2018**, *3*, 5. [CrossRef]
51. Stankiewicz, J.M.; Weiner, H.L. An argument for broad use of high efficacy treatments in early multiple sclerosis. *Neurol. Neuroimmunol. Neuroinflamm.* **2019**, *7*, e636. [CrossRef] [PubMed]
52. Comi, G. Induction vs. escalating therapy in Multiple Sclerosis: Practical implications. *Neurol. Sci.* **2008**, *29*, 253–255. [CrossRef]
53. Fenu, G.; Lorefice, L.; Frau, F.; Coghe, G.; Marrosu, M.; Cocco, E. Induction and escalation therapies in multiple sclerosis. *Anti-Inflamm. Anti-Allergy Agents Med. Chem.* **2015**, *14*, 26–34. [CrossRef]
54. Rieckmann, P. Concepts of induction and escalation therapy in multiple sclerosis. *J. Neurol. Sci.* **2009**, *277*, S42–S45. [CrossRef]
55. Wingerchuk, D.M.; Carter, J.L. Multiple Sclerosis: Current and Emerging Disease-Modifying Therapies and Treatment Strategies. *Mayo Clin. Proc.* **2014**, *89*, 225–240. [CrossRef]
56. Freedman, M.S. Induction vs. escalation of therapy for relapsing Multiple Sclerosis: The evidence. *Neurol. Sci.* **2008**, *29*, 250–252. [CrossRef] [PubMed]
57. Coyle, P.K. Commentary: The Multiple Sclerosis Controversy: Is It Escalation or Induction High Efficacy? *Neurotherapeutics* **2020**, *17*, 971–972. [CrossRef]
58. Buron, M.D.; Chalmer, T.A.; Sellebjerg, F.; Barzinji, I.; Christensen, J.R.; Christensen, M.K.; Hansen, V.; Illes, Z.; Jensen, H.B.; Kant, M.; et al. Initial high-efficacy disease-modifying therapy in multiple sclerosis. *Neurology* **2020**, *95*, e1041–e1051. [CrossRef]

59. Harding, K.; Williams, O.; Willis, M.; Hrastelj, J.; Rimmer, A.; Joseph, F.; Tomassini, V.; Wardle, M.; Pickersgill, T.; Robertson, N.; et al. Clinical Outcomes of Escalation vs Early Intensive Disease-Modifying Therapy in Patients with Multiple Sclerosis. *JAMA Neurol.* **2019**, *76*, 536–541. [CrossRef]
60. He, A.; Merkel, B.; Brown, W.; Ryerson, L.Z.; Kister, I.; Malpas, C.B.; Sharmin, S.; Horakova, D.; Havrdova, E.K.; Spelman, T.; et al. Timing of high-efficacy therapy for multiple sclerosis: A retrospective observational cohort study. *Lancet Neurol.* **2020**, *19*, 307–316. [CrossRef]
61. Iaffaldano, P.; Lucisano, G.; Caputo, F.; Paolicelli, D.; Patti, F.; Zaffaroni, M.; Morra, V.B.; Pozzilli, C.; De Luca, G.; Inglese, M.; et al. Long-term disability trajectories in relapsing multiple sclerosis patients treated with early intensive or escalation treatment strategies. *Ther. Adv. Neurol. Disord.* **2021**, *14*, 17562864211019574. [CrossRef]
62. Prosperini, L.; Mancinelli, C.R.; Solaro, C.M.; Nociti, V.; Haggiag, S.; Cordioli, C.; De Giglio, L.; De Rossi, N.; Galgani, S.; Rasia, S.; et al. Induction Versus Escalation in Multiple Sclerosis: A 10-Year Real World Study. *Neurotherapeutics* **2020**, *17*, 994–1004. [CrossRef] [PubMed]
63. Merkel, B.; Butzkueven, H.; Traboulsee, A.L.; Havrdova, E.K.; Kalincik, T. Timing of high-efficacy therapy in relapsing-remitting multiple sclerosis: A systematic review. *Autoimmun. Rev.* **2017**, *16*, 658–665. [CrossRef] [PubMed]
64. Le Page, E.; Edan, G. Induction or escalation therapy for patients with multiple sclerosis? *Rev. Neurol.* **2018**, *174*, 449–457. [CrossRef]
65. Horáková, D.; Boster, A.; Bertolotto, A.; Freedman, M.S.; Firmino, I.; Cavalier, S.J.; Jacobs, A.K.; Thangavelu, K.; Daizadeh, N.; Poole, E.M.; et al. Proportion of alemtuzumab-treated patients converting from relapsing-remitting multiple sclerosis to secondary progressive multiple sclerosis over 6 years. *Mult. Scler. J. Exp. Transl. Clin.* **2020**, *6*, 2055217320972137. [CrossRef]
66. Kalincik, T.; Brown, W.; Robertson, N.; Willis, M.; Scolding, N.; Rice, C.; Wilkins, A.; Pearson, O.; Ziemssen, T.; Hutchinson, M.; et al. Treatment effectiveness of alemtuzumab compared with natalizumab, fingolimod, and interferon beta in relapsing-remitting multiple sclerosis: A cohort study. *Lancet Neurol.* **2017**, *16*, 271–281. [CrossRef]
67. Granqvist, M.; Boremalm, M.; Poorghobad, A.; Svenningsson, A.; Salzer, J.; Frisell, T.; Piehl, F. Comparative Effectiveness of Rituximab and Other Initial Treatment Choices for Multiple Sclerosis. *JAMA Neurol.* **2018**, *75*, 320–327. [CrossRef]
68. Casanova, B.; Jarque, I.; Gascón, F.; Hernández-Boluda, J.C.; Pérez-Miralles, F.; De La Rubia, J.; Alcalá, C.; Sanz, J.; Mallada, J.; Cervelló, A.; et al. Autologous hematopoietic stem cell transplantation in relapsing-remitting multiple sclerosis: Comparison with secondary progressive multiple sclerosis. *Neurol. Sci.* **2017**, *38*, 1213–1221. [CrossRef] [PubMed]
69. Simonsen, C.S.; Flemmen, H.Ø.; Broch, L.; Brunborg, C.; Berg-Hansen, P.; Moen, S.M.; Celius, E.G. Early High Efficacy Treatment in Multiple Sclerosis Is the Best Predictor of Future Disease Activity Over 1 and 2 Years in a Norwegian Population-Based Registry. *Front. Neurol.* **2021**, *12*, 1009. [CrossRef] [PubMed]

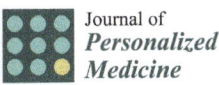

Article

Assessing Blood-Based Biomarkers to Define a Therapeutic Window for Natalizumab

Júlia Granell-Geli [1,2], Cristina Izquierdo-Gracia [3], Ares Sellés-Rius [1], Aina Teniente-Serra [1,2], Silvia Presas-Rodríguez [3], María José Mansilla [1,2], Luis Brieva [4], Javier Sotoca [5], María Alba Mañé-Martínez [6], Ester Moral [7], Irene Bragado [3], Susan Goelz [8], Eva Martínez-Cáceres [1,2,*,†] and Cristina Ramo-Tello [3,*,†]

1. Division of Immunology, LCMN Hospital Universitari Germans Trias i Pujol and Research Institute, Campus Can Ruti, 08916 Badalona, Spain; juliagranellgeli@gmail.com (J.G.-G.); aselles@igtp.cat (A.S.-R.); ateniente@igtp.cat (A.T.-S.); mjmansilla@igtp.cat (M.J.M.)
2. Department of Cellular Biology, Physiology and Immunology, Universitat Autònoma de Barcelona, 08193 Bellaterra, Spain
3. Multiple Sclerosis Unit, Department of Neurosciences, Hospital Universitari Germans Trias i Pujol, 08916 Badalona, Spain; cizquierdogr.germanstrias@gencat.cat (C.I.-G.); spresas@igtp.cat (S.P.-R.); ibragado@csap.cat (I.B.)
4. Multiple Sclerosis Unit, Hospital Universitari Arnau de Vilanova, 25198 Lleida, Spain; lbrieva.lleida.ics@gencat.cat
5. Neurology Service, Hospital Universitari Mútua Terrassa, 08221 Terrassa, Spain; jsotoca@vhebron.net
6. Neurology Service, Hospital Universitari Joan XXIII, Universitat Rovira i Virgili, 43005 Tarragona, Spain; amane.hj23.ics@gencat.cat
7. Multiple Sclerosis Unit, Hospital Sant Joan Despí Moisès Broggi, 08970 Sant Joan Despí, Spain; ester.moral@sanitatintegral.org
8. Biogen Idec, Cambridge, MA 02142, USA; segoelz@gmail.com
* Correspondence: emmartinez.germanstrias@gencat.cat (E.M.-C.); cramot.germanstrias@gencat.cat (C.R.-T.)
† Shared senior co-authorship.

Abstract: Natalizumab is a monoclonal antibody that binds CD49d. Although it is one of the most effective treatments for Relapsing-Remitting Multiple Sclerosis (RRMS), a dosing regimen has not been optimized for safety and efficacy in individual patients. We aimed to identify biomarkers to monitor Natalizumab treatment and to establish a personalized dose utilizing an ongoing longitudinal study in 29 RRMS patients under Natalizumab with standard interval dose (SD) of 300 mg/4 wks or extended interval dose (EID) of 300 mg/6 wks. Blood samples were analyzed by flow cytometry to determine CD49d saturation and expression in several T and B lymphocytes subpopulations. Each patient was analyzed at two different timepoints separated by 3 Natalizumab administrations. Natalizumab and sVCAM-1 levels in serum were also analyzed using ELISA. To determine the reproducibility of various markers, two different timepoints were compared and no significant differences were observed for CD49d expression nor for saturation; SD patients had higher saturation levels (~80%) than EID patients (~60%). A positive correlation exists between CD49d saturation and Natalizumab serum levels. CD49d expression and saturation are stable parameters that could be used as biomarkers in the immunomonitoring of Natalizumab treatment. Moreover, Natalizumab and sVCAM-1 serum levels could be used to optimize an individual's dosing schedule.

Keywords: multiple sclerosis; natalizumab; extended interval dose; biomarker; CD49d; sVCAM-1; immunomonitoring; personalized dose

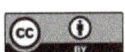

1. Introduction

Natalizumab (NTZ) is a humanized IgG4κ monoclonal antibody that selectively binds by allosteric antagonism to α4-integrin (CD49d), preventing leukocyte migration into the central nervous system (CNS) in multiple sclerosis (MS) patients [1]. α4-integrins form heterodimers with β-subunits [β1 (CD29) and β7] to form functional molecules [2]. α4β1 (VLA-4) and α4β7 are located on leukocytes surface and interact with VCAM-1 and MAdCAM-1, respectively, for the firm adhesion of leukocytes to endothelial cells, a necessary step for leukocyte extravasation into the inflamed tissue.

The interaction of VLA-4 with VCAM-1 not only facilitates adhesion of leukocytes to the endothelium enabling the transmigration of circulating leukocytes across the blood-brain barrier (BBB) [3,4], but also can increase the activation and proliferation of lymphocytes [5,6]. This process leads to a cascade of local chemokines and cytokines that activates more lymphocytes and further promotes adhesion and transmigration of immune cells into the inflamed tissue [7,8]. In addition, pro-inflammatory factors released in autoimmune conditions such as MS can increase the expression of VCAM-1 on the endothelial cell surface allowing leukocyte binding to the BBB which, in turn, promotes the release as soluble VCAM-1 (sVCAM-1) [9]. This suggests that serum levels of sVCAM-1 could be a marker of immune cells binding to the endothelial barrier as well as endothelial barrier activity.

NTZ is generally administered intravenously at 300 mg every 4 weeks in relapsing-remitting MS (RRMS) patients. Although it is one of the most effective treatments [10] its use is associated with a very severe side effect, the risk of developing Progressive Multifocal Leukoencephalopathy (PML) [11]. PML is an uncommon and severe opportunistic brain infection caused by the reactivation of the neurotropic John Cunningham virus (JCV), as a consequence of immunosurveillance debilitation [10,12]. JCV is present in ~50–70% of the population [13], as evidenced by the presence of anti-JCV antibodies in serum. It may remain asymptomatic throughout life, being generally considered as non-pathogenic [14,15]. However, it can become neurotropic and cause PML and demyelination of axons as a consequence of lytic infection of the myelin-producing oligodendrocytes. The prognosis for PML is often bleak, with a high fatality rate [13]. Though it is extremely rare (only 0.2 per 100,000 of the general population) [13], the PML risk becomes significant when a patient is immune compromised or is treated with a therapy that can inhibit CNS immune surveillance such as NTZ.

One approach to reduce the risk of PML is to define the lowest efficacious dose for an individual patient; the premise being that this would also be the safest dose. The standard dosing of 300 mg every 4 weeks maintains a maximal VLA-4 saturation, defined as >80% saturation of these receptors on PBMCs [16]. The extended dosage of NTZ is an attempt to define the saturation level of VLA-4 that maintains the clinical effectiveness of the drug but allows a slightest increase in CNS immunosurveillance in order to reduce PML risk [17]. It has been reported that patients positive for anti-JCV antibodies receiving NTZ in extended interval dose (EID) appear to have a lower risk of PML compared with those with the standard dose (SD) [18].

In this study, we aimed to identify biomarkers to monitor NTZ treatment and to establish a personalized dose in NTZ-treated patients. Unlike previous studies where PBMCs were used, we have validated CD49d saturation and expression on T-cells (CD4$^+$ and CD8$^+$) and B-cells to be used as biomarkers to monitor and personalize the treatment by two different protocols. We have also explored the use of sVCAM-1 in serum as a biomarker to monitor MS disease activity. In addition, we have studied the correlation between CD49d saturation and NTZ levels in serum.

2. Materials and Methods

2.1. Study Design

This is a pilot, multicentric, prospective, open study in RRMS patients treated with NTZ, performed in the Multiple Sclerosis Unit of the Hospital Germans Trias i Pujol (Badalona), the Hospital Mútua de Terrassa (Terrassa), the Hospital Arnau de Vilanova (Lleida), the Hospital de Sant Joan Despí Moisès Broggi, the Hospital Joan XXIII (Tarragona), and the Hospital de Mataró.

Expanded disability scale score (EDSS) and annualized relapse rate (ARR) were obtained during clinical visits. Patients under NTZ treatment from 18 years old were included in the study and were classified in 2 groups. The first group included patients under intravenous NTZ treatment that were clinically or radiologically active in SD of 300 mg/4 wks with at least 13 uninterrupted doses. The second group included patients under NTZ treatment for at least 6 months in EID of 300 mg/6 wks that were clinically or radiologically active (Active) or remained clinically and radiologically stable (Inactive). Clinically active patients were defined as those who presented a relapse at some point under Natalizumab treatment, and as radiologically active patients those who presented at least two new lesions in T2 brain MRI sequences or one new gadolinium lesion at some point during the treatment, but not specifically during our study.

The assignment of each patient to a specific therapeutic strategy was previous and independent regarding the participation of the patient to the study. According to our daily clinical practice, all patients started the treatment with Natalizumab in SD and after 13 infusions it was proposed to switch to EID if they did not have clinical and radiological activity. Whether patients showed clinical or radiological activity, they remained in SD schedule. Blood samples were obtained before every NTZ infusion in a first timepoint (V1) and a second timepoint after 3 NTZ administrations (V2). A total of 30 mL of peripheral blood were extracted by venipuncture (10 mL in a serum-separator tube and 20 mL of whole blood in EDTA tube). All patients gave written informed consent to participate in the study and approval was obtained from the corresponding local Ethic Committees.

Patients who had planned to withdraw NTZ treatment during the period of the study, who will not be able to comply with the study procedures, having suffered a relapse during the 30 days prior to the baseline visit, or an infection that had required more than symptomatic treatment during the 30 days prior to the baseline visit were excluded from the study.

2.2. Flow Cytometry

Whole blood samples were collected in EDTA tubes, kept at room temperature, and processed within the next 24 h. Several parameters were analyzed in peripheral blood by multiparametric flow cytometry by two different protocols performed in parallel.

2.2.1. Whole Blood Analysis

Quantification of CD49d and bound NTZ molecules was performed by Quantitative Flow Cytometry on T ($CD4^+$ and $CD8^+$) and B ($CD19^+$) lymphocytes following a protocol set in our lab [19]. Tracking and calibration of the flow cytometer was performed using Rainbow 6 Peak calibration particles and QuantiBRITE phycoerythrin (PE) beads (BD Bioscience, Franklin Lakes, NJ, USA) before sample acquisition. Briefly, 5 mL of peripheral blood were lysed with non-fixing ammonium chloride-based lysing reagent (FACSLysing Solution®, BD) for 10 min. A total of 100,000 cells per tube were incubated 1 or 2 times (depending on the labelling) for 20 min at room temperature with pre-titrated amounts of the monoclonal antibodies anti-CD3 V450 (clone UCHT1, BD), anti-CD4 FITC (clone SK3, BD), anti-CD8 APC-H7 (clone SK1, BD), anti-CD19 PerCP-Cy5.5 (clone SJ25C1, BD), and either anti-CD49d (clone 9F10, BD) or huIgG4 Fc PE (clone HP6025, Southern Biotech) to measure bound NTZ. After two washes with PBS, lymphocytes were acquired on a FACSCanto II flow cytometer (BD Bioscience), and all samples were analyzed with FACSDiva software (BD Bioscience) (see analysis in Figure A1). In parallel, a Fluorescence Minus-One (FMO) was performed, for each sample, to establish a cut-off between the negative and the positive populations for huIgG4 and CD49d fluorescence signal. Quantification of huIgG4 and CD49d surface molecules was performed according to the instructions of QuantiBRITE manufacturer. The molecules per cell surface were obtained by linear regression, and the CD49d receptor occupancy (RO) was calculated as the percentage of NTZ bound to CD49d with the following formula: [(bound NTZ molecules)/(total CD49d molecules)] × 100.

2.2.2. PBMCs Analysis

A total of 15 mL of peripheral blood were diluted with PBS and PBMCs were isolated by Ficoll-Paque Plus (density 1.077. GE Healthcare). After 2 washes, PBMCs were distributed into wells of 96-well plate (100,000 cells/well). Cells were first incubated with an Fc Block for 20 min at 4 °C and washed. Then they were incubated for 30 min at 4 °C with the corresponding amount of the monoclonal antibodies anti-IgD FITC (clone IA6-2, BD), anti-CD45RA PerCP-Cy5.5 (clone HI100, Biolegend), anti-CD197 (CCR7) BV421 (clone G043H7, Biolegend), anti-CD19 BV510 (clone HIB19, Biolegend), anti-CD49d BV711 (clone 9F10, Biolegend), anti-CD3 BV605 (clone SK7, BD), NTZ-AF647 APC (Biogen), anti-Integrin β1 (CD29) Alexa700 (clone TS2/16, Biolegend), anti-CD8 APC-H7 (clone SK1, BD), anti-Integrin β7 PE (clone FIB504, Biolegend), anti-CD27 PE-CF594 (clone M-T271, BD), anti-CD4 PE-Cy7 (clone OKT4, Biolegend). After two washes with PBSA, lymphocytes were acquired on a LSRFortessa flow cytometer (BD Bioscience), and all samples were analyzed with FlowJo software (BD Bioscience) (see analysis in Figure A2). UltraComp eBeadsTM Compensation Beads (ThermoFisher, Waltham, MA, USA) were used to compensate each individual fluorochrome. FMO was performed for each sample to establish a cut-off between the negative and the positive populations for CD49d, NTZ-AF647, CD29 and α7-Integrin fluorescence signal.

The acquired and analyzed subpopulations were $CD4^+CD27^+$, $CD4^+CCR7^+CD45^+$ (Naive), $CD4^+CCR7^+CD45^-$ (Central Memory (CM)), $CD4^+CCR7^-CD45^-$ (Effector Memory (EM)), $CD4^+CCR7^-CD45^+$ (Effector), $CD8^+CD27^+$, $CD8^+CCR7^+CD45^+$ (Naive), $CD8^+CCR7^+CD45^-$ (CM), $CD8^+CCR7^-CD45^-$ (EM), $CD8^+CCR7^-CD45^+$ (Effector), $CD19^+CD27^-IgD^+$ (Naive), $CD19^+CD27^+IgD^-$ (Switched), $CD19^+CD27^+IgD^+$ (Non-switched), $CD19^+CD27^-IgD^-$ (Double Negative (DN)).

2.3. Serum Analysis

A total of 4 mL of serum contained in 10 mL serum-separator tubes were frozen at −80 °C for the determination of NTZ and sVCAM-1 levels in both first and second extractions.

NTZ was quantified using an ELISA method with a mouse anti-human IgG4 (Fc-HRP, Southern Biotech). Briefly, Coating Material (12C4, Tysabri anti-ID) was diluted from 2 mg/mL to 1.0 µg/mL in PBS and 100 µL of 1.0 µg/mL coating solution was added to each well and incubated overnight at 2 to 8 °C shaking at 400 rpm. After washing, 300 µL of Blocking Buffer (Thermo Scientific) was added to each well, and the plate incubated for 2 h at ambient room temperature (ART) while shaking at 400 rpm. Controls and samples were thawed and diluted at least 1/50. After washing, 100 µL of diluted controls and samples were added and incubated for 1 h at ART on plate shaker set to 400 rpm. Plate was washed 3 times and dried, and 100 µL of detection solution (1/20,000 in Casein) was added to each well and incubated for 30 min at ART on plate shaker set to 400 rpm. Finally, the plate was washed 3 times and dried, and 100 µL of TMB Substrate (Thermo Scientific) were added to each well and incubated at ART approximately for 5 min. Substrate reaction was stopped by adding 100 µL of Stop Solution (1N H2SO4, Fisher) to each well and plate reading was done within approximately 15 min of stopping the reaction using the microplate reader set to 450 nm. Standard curve was prepared in Assay buffer (2% Human Serum in Casein).

Analysis of soluble human VCAM-1 was performed following the instructions of DuoSet® ELISA Development system manufacturer.

2.4. Statistical Analysis

To test the stability of these parameters over time, first and second extractions were compared separately for each group (SD and EID) using Two-tailed paired t-test. The obtained values were compared between treatment groups for both first and second extraction using Two-tailed unpaired t-test. Two-tailed p values < 0.05 were considered statistically significant.

Correlation test was performed by comparing CD49d saturation levels and NTZ serum levels for the first extraction ($n = 20$) and second extraction ($n = 14$). Two-tailed p values < 0.05 were considered statistically significant.

All statistical analysis were performed using GraphPad Prism software (version 8.4.0; La Jolla, CA, USA).

3. Results

A total of 29 RRMS patients (72.4% females) under NTZ treatment with mean age of 44.4 ± 10.5 years and body mass index of 23.3 ± 3.6 participated in the study and were classified in 2 groups. The first group included 8 active patients (27.58%) in SD. The second group included 21 patients in EID, of which 19 patients (65.6%) were inactive and 2 patients (6.89%) were active. Demographic and clinical features of the patients are represented in Table 1.

Table 1. Demographic and clinical features of the 29 RRMS patients of the study.

Demographic and Clinical Features	All (n = 29)	Active		Inactive EID (n = 19)
		SD (n = 8)	EID (n = 2)	
Age, mean (SD)	44 (10.5)	36.5 (9.5)	59.5 (3.5)	46 (9)
Gender (F), n (%)	21 (72.4)	5 (62.5)	2 (100)	14 (73.6)
BMI, mean (SD)	23.3 (3.6)	22 (2.7)	21.2 (2.2)	24 (4)
Serology JCV (+), n (%)	4 (13.8)	2 (20)	1 (50)	1 (5.2)
Time since diagnosis (y), mean (SD)	13.5 (7.3)	10.2 (8.2)	23 (9.9)	13.9 (6)
Time under NTZ (y), mean (SD)	7.3 (3.7)	7.3 (2.3)	11.5 (3.5)	11.2 (3.3)
➤ Under NTZ in EID	-	-	3.5 (3.5)	6.8 (2.8)
Previous treatment, n (%)	21 (72.4)	5 (62.5)	2 (100)	14 (73.6)
Activity under NTZ, n (%)				
➤ Relapse	8 (27.5)	6 (75)	2 (100)	-
➤ MRI activity	6 (20.6)	6 (75)	0	-
EDSS, mean (SD)	3.2 (1.9)	2.9 (2.2)	4.3 (2.5)	3.2 (1.8)

BMI: body mass index; EDSS: Expanded Disability Status Scale; EID: extended interval dose; F: female; JCV: John Cunningham virus; MRI: magnetic resonance imaging; NTZ: natalizumab; SD: standard desviation; y: years.

3.1. CD49d Is a Good Biomarker to Monitor Natalizumab Treatment

The aim of this analysis was to assess if CD49d expression could be used as a putative biomarker to monitor the efficacy of NTZ treatment in RRMS patients.

First, we checked whether the expression levels were stable over time by comparing the two timepoints (V1 and V2) for both SD and EID patients in all T and B cell subpopulations. CD49d surface molecules and bound NTZ (Figure 1a–c) as well as CD49d saturation (Figure 1d) were determined by Quantitative Flow Cytometry in whole blood in 29 patients receiving NTZ therapy (SD, $n = 8$; EID, $n = 21$). None of the lymphocyte subpopulations showed significant differences between V1 and V2 for any of these biomarkers except for the bound NTZ levels in both $CD4^+$ and $CD8^+$ T cell subpopulations (Figure 1b) and the CD49d saturation in $CD4^+$ cells in patients receiving NTZ in SD (Figure 1d).

In parallel with the measurement of CD49d saturation, an alternative flow cytometry panel was performed in PBMCs to assess the percentage of positive cells for CD49d. $CD4^+$ Effector cells were excluded from this analysis as there were very few cells to define the positive population for each marker and then to draw a consistent conclusion about their percentage of expression. No significant differences were observed between V1 and V2 in CD49d expression for any of the studied lymphocyte subsets for this marker (Figure 2).

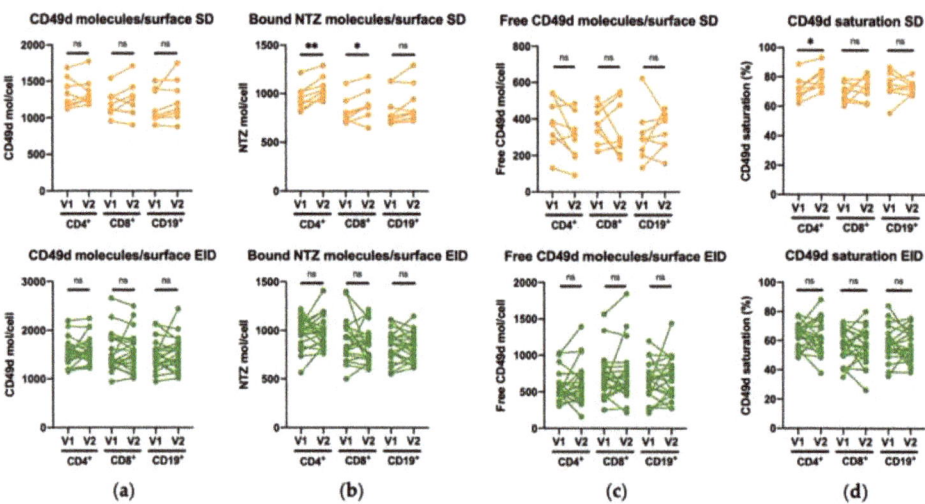

Figure 1. Comparison between the first extraction (V1) and the second extraction (V2) within CD4$^+$ and CD8$^+$ T lymphocytes, and CD19$^+$ B lymphocytes for the CD49d surface molecules levels and saturation percentage in RRMS patients under Natalizumab treatment in SD or EID. Mean of (**a**) CD49d molecules/cell surface, (**b**) bound NTZ/cell surface, (**c**) free CD49d molecules/cell surface, and (**d**) CD49d saturation percentage in CD4$^+$ and CD8$^+$ T lymphocytes, and CD19$^+$ B lymphocytes in the SD (n = 8) and EID (n = 21) groups. Each dot represents the number of PE molecules per cell for each patient in either V1 and V2, translated into the levels of the corresponding antibodies (anti-CD49d PE and huIgG4 Fc PE). EID, extended interval dosing; NTZ, natalizumab; SD, standard dosing. ns: $p > 0.05$, * $p < 0.05$, ** $p < 0.01$.

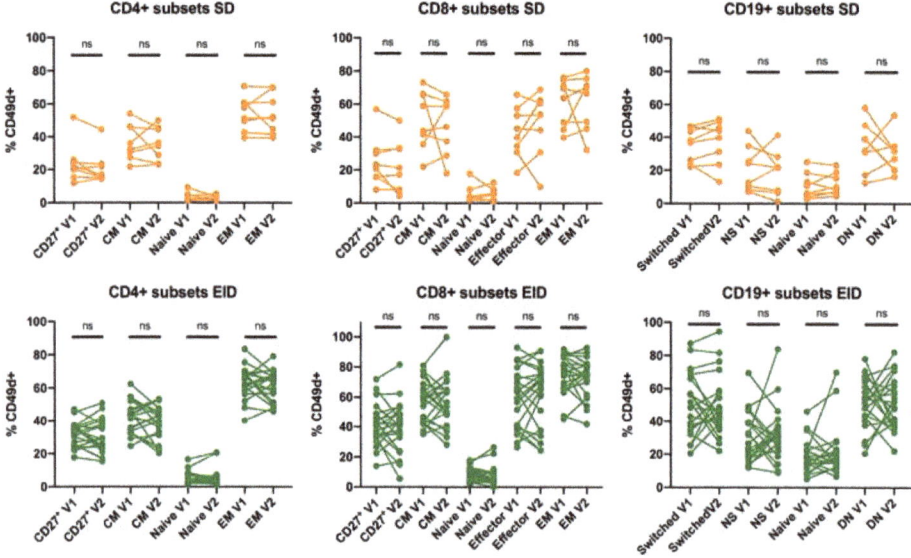

Figure 2. Comparison of first (V1) and second (V2) extractions within CD4$^+$ and CD8$^+$ T lymphocytes, and CD19$^+$ B lymphocytes subpopulations in RRMS patients under Natalizumab treatment in SD or EID. Percentage of expression of in several CD4$^+$ and CD8$^+$ T lymphocytes, and CD19$^+$ B lymphocytes subsets. Each dot represents the percentage of expression for each marker regarding their parent population (CD4$^+$ or CD8$^+$ T lymphocytes, or CD19$^+$ B lymphocytes populations) in the SD (n = 8) and EID (n = 21) groups. CM, Central Memory; DN, Double Negative; EID, extended interval dosing; EM, Effector Memory; NS, Non-Switched; NTZ, natalizumab; SD, standard dosing. ns: $p > 0.05$.

3.2. Extended Interval Dosing Reduces CD49d Saturation

Once the stability of CD49d saturation and expression were assessed, the differences between SD and EID groups were studied to test whether differential CD49d values could be defined. The mean (V1 and V2) of CD49d molecules per cell surface in lymphocyte subpopulations measured in whole blood was lower in patients treated with NTZ in SD schedule compared with the ones in EID (CD4$^+$ CD49d molecules/cell surface: 1334 vs. 1535; CD8$^+$ CD49d molecules/cell surface: 1191 vs. 1558; CD19$^+$ CD49d molecules/cell surface: 1158 vs. 1475) (Figure 3a). Conversely, no significant differences in the mean of NTZ bound molecules per cell surface in lymphocyte subpopulations was observed between SD and EID groups (CD4$^+$ NTZ molecules/cell surface: 956.9 vs. 970.9; CD8$^+$ NTZ molecules/cell surface: 819.6 vs. 895.7; CD19$^+$ NTZ molecules/cell surface: 848.4 vs. 841.3) (Figure 3b). As a result of this lower number of CD49d molecules in SD patients, together with the same levels of bound NTZ in both groups, the percentage of CD49d saturation was higher in SD patients compared with EID patients (CD4$^+$ CD49d% saturation: 72.31 vs. 63.82; CD8$^+$ CD49d% saturation: 68.97 vs. 55.91; CD19$^+$ CD49d% saturation: 73.74 vs. 58.30) (Figure 3d). In addition, we also checked the amount of free CD49d as a verification with the following formula: *(total CD49d molecules) − (bound NTZ molecules)*. As expected, mean of free CD49d molecules per cell surface in lymphocytes subpopulations was lower in SD patients than EID patients (CD4$^+$ free CD49d molecules/cell surface: 376.6 vs. 564.0; CD8$^+$ free CD49d molecules/cell surface: 371.8 vs. 697.9; CD19$^+$ free CD49d molecules/cell surface: 309.3 vs. 634.0) (Figure 3c). The data represented here corresponds to the first extraction (V1), but similar results were also obtained for the second extraction (V2) (Figure A3).

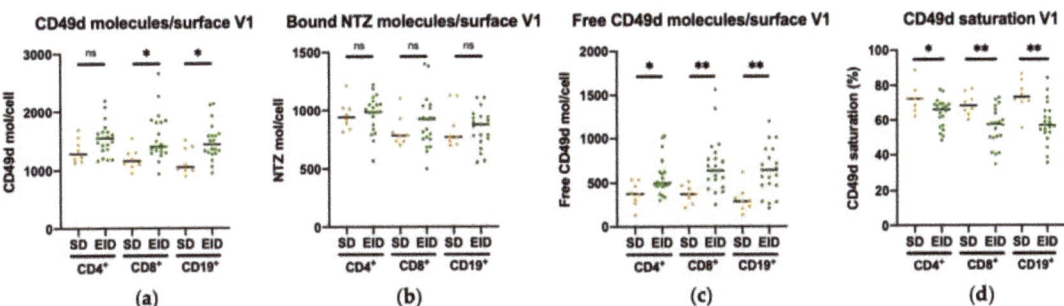

Figure 3. CD49d surface molecules levels and saturation percentage in CD4$^+$ and CD8$^+$ T lymphocytes, and CD19$^+$ B lymphocytes in RRMS patients under Natalizumab treatment in SD or EID. Mean of (**a**) CD49d molecules/cell surface, (**b**) bound NTZ/cell surface, (**c**) free CD49d molecules/cell surface, and (**d**) CD49d saturation percentage in CD4$^+$ and CD8$^+$ T lymphocytes, and CD19$^+$ B lymphocytes in the SD ($n = 8$) and EID ($n = 21$) groups. Each dot represents the number of PE molecules per cell for each patient in the first extraction (V1), translated into the levels of the corresponding antibodies (anti-CD49d PE and huIgG4 Fc PE). EID, extended interval dosing; NTZ, natalizumab; SD, standard dosing. Ns: $p > 0.05$, * $p < 0.05$, ** $p < 0.01$.

We then aimed to check whether there were significant differences between SD and EID patients in CD49d expression in PBMCs for any of the subsets to define which subpopulations showed differences in the expression of the markers due to the dosing schedule. That would allow us to establish some reference values or range of values for each group in order to monitor the patients and to have a criterion to decide their dosing schedule should be altered. SD and EID groups were compared for both the first (V1) and the second (V2) extractions separately. Significant differences between SD and EID were observed in CD8$^+$ CD27$^+$ (Figure 4a) and CD19$^+$ DN (Figure 4b) for CD49d expression. Several additional subsets also showed significant differences in V1 or V2 (Figures A4 and A5), while the rest of subsets did not (Table 2).

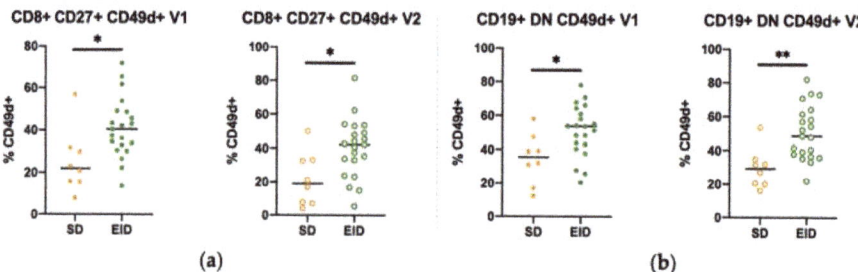

Figure 4. Representation of SD and EID groups in some $CD4^+$ and $CD8^+$ T lymphocytes, and $CD19^+$ B lymphocytes subpopulations in RRMS patients under Natalizumab treatment in both first (V1) and second (V2) extractions. Percentage of expression of CD49d in (**a**) $CD8^+CD27^+$ T lymphocytes and (**b**) $CD19^+$ DN B lymphocytes. Each dot represents the percentage of expression for each marker regarding their parent population ($CD4^+$ or $CD8^+$ T lymphocytes, or $CD19^+$ B lymphocytes populations) in the SD (*n* = 8) or EID (*n* = 21) groups. DN, Double Negative; EID, extended interval dosing; NTZ, natalizumab; SD, standard dosing. Ns: $p > 0.05$, * $p < 0.05$, ** $p < 0.01$.

Table 2. Summary table of the most relevant cell-surface and serum markers analysed.

Marker	Lymphocyte Subset	SD vs. EID	Stability (V1 vs. V2)
Total CD49d	$CD4^+$ $CD8^+$ $CD19^+$	1334 vs. 1535 1191 vs. 1558 1158 vs. 1475	Good
CD49d saturation (%)	$CD4^+$ $CD8^+$ $CD19^+$	72.31 vs. 63.82 68.97 vs. 55.91 73.74 vs. 58.30	Good
% CD49d	$CD8^+\ CD27^+$ $CD19^+$ DN	25.24 vs. 41.20 34.58 vs. 50.94	Good Good
CD29	All subpopulations		Poor
β7-Integrin	All subpopulations		Good
NTZ serum (ng/mL)	-	47814 vs. 12490	Marginal
sVCAM-1 (pg/mL)	-	69341 vs. 97955	Good

DN: double negative; EID: extended interval dose; NTZ: natalizumab; SD: standard dose; sVCAM-1: soluble vascular cell adhesion molecule-1; V1/V2: visit 1/visit 2.

3.3. CD29 and β7-Integrin Are Not Good Biomarkers to Monitor Natalizumab Treatment

In parallel with the study of CD49d saturation and expression, other surface molecules were studied as putative biomarkers to monitor NTZ treatment in PBMCs of RRMS patients. The percentage of positive cells for CD29 and β7-integrin was determined regarding all $CD4^+$ and $CD8^+$ T and $CD19^+$ B lymphocytes subpopulations. $CD4^+$ Effector cells were excluded from this analysis as there were very few cells to define the positive population for each marker and then to draw a consistent conclusion about their percentage of expression. First, the stability of the expression levels of these markers over time was checked by comparing the two timepoints (V1 and V2) for both SD and EID patients in all T and B cell subsets.

No significant differences were observed between V1 and V2 in any of the studied lymphocyte subsets for β7-integrin (Figure A6). Conversely, CD29 showed significant differences between extractions (V1 vs. V2) in some lymphocyte subsets for both SD and EID groups (Figure 5).

The β7-Integrin was further studied by comparing the SD and EID groups for all $CD4^+$ and $CD8^+$ T and $CD19^+$ B lymphocytes subpopulations to assess whether it could work as a biomarker. None of the studied subsets showed significant differences between SD and EID groups.

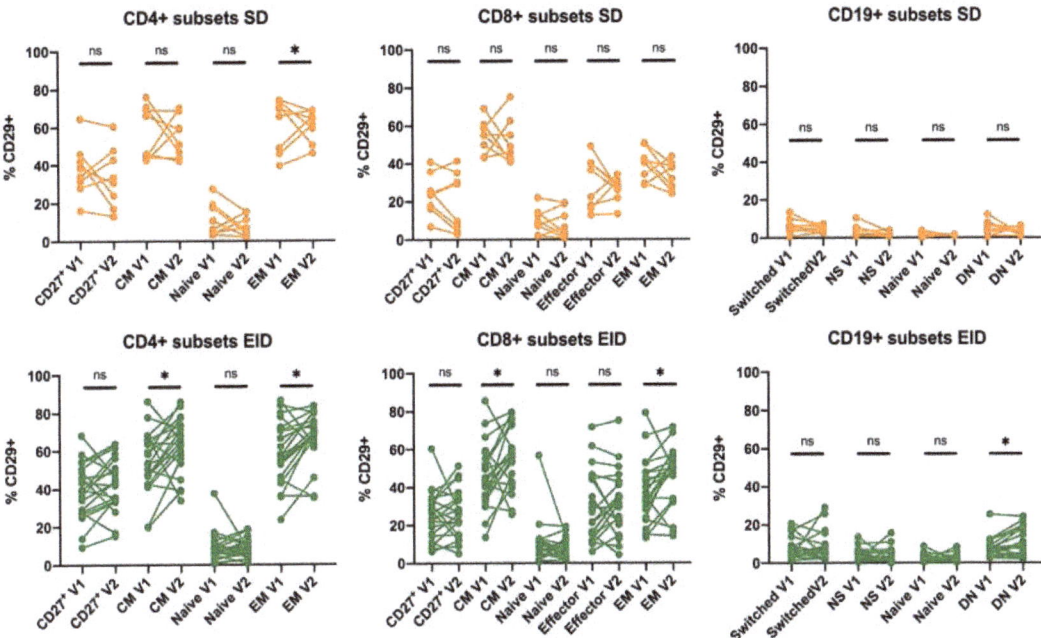

Figure 5. Comparison of first (V1) and second (V2) extractions within CD4$^+$ and CD8$^+$ T lymphocytes, and CD19$^+$ B lymphocytes subpopulations in RRMS patients under Natalizumab treatment in SD or EID. Percentage of expression of CD29 in all CD4$^+$ and CD8$^+$ T lymphocytes, and CD19$^+$ B lymphocytes subsets. Each dot represents the percentage of expression of CD29 regarding their parent population (CD4$^+$ or CD8$^+$ T lymphocytes, or CD19$^+$ B lymphocytes populations) in the SD ($n = 8$) and EID ($n = 21$) groups. CM, Central Memory; DN, Double Negative; EID, extended interval dosing; EM, Effector Memory; NS, Non-Switched; SD, standard dosing. Ns: $p > 0.05$, * $p < 0.05$.

3.4. Natalizumab and sVCAM-1 Are Putative Serum Biomarkers to Monitor the Treatment

Several markers in serum were also analyzed to study whether they could be useful for the monitoring of the NTZ treatment. We had the opportunity to analyze 21 patients (SD $n = 7$ and EID $n = 14$), of which 15 patients (EID $n = 9$, SD $n = 6$) were analyzed for both first (V1) and second (V2) extractions.

First, V1 and V2 were compared to check the stability of NTZ and sVCAM-1 over time in both SD and EID groups. All conditions appeared to be stable over time except for the NTZ levels in SD condition and this may be due to the low number of subjects in this group (Figure 6).

After checking the stability of these markers, SD and EID groups were compared to study if there were significant differences for the levels of these serum parameters. Here we show the results for the first extraction as an example, as the sample size is higher than the for the second extraction. The levels of NTZ were significantly higher in SD patients than in EID patients (Figure 7a), while the levels of sVCAM-1 were significantly lower in SD patients compared with EID patients (Figure 7b).

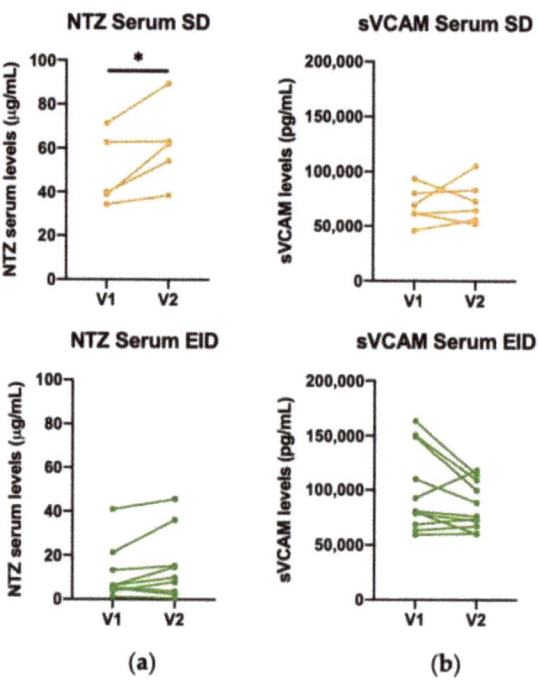

Figure 6. Comparison of V1 and V2 for NTZ and sVCAM in serum in RRMS patients under Natalizumab treatment in SD or EID. Levels of (**a**) NTZ (μg/mL) and (**b**) sVCAM (pg/mL) in serum in the SD ($n = 6$) and EID ($n = 9$) groups. Each dot represents the concentration of NTZ or sVCAM in serum for each patient in either the first extraction (V1) and the second extraction (V2). EID, extended interval dosing; NTZ, natalizumab; SD, standard dosing; sVCAM, soluble VCAM. ns: $p > 0.05$, * $p < 0.05$.

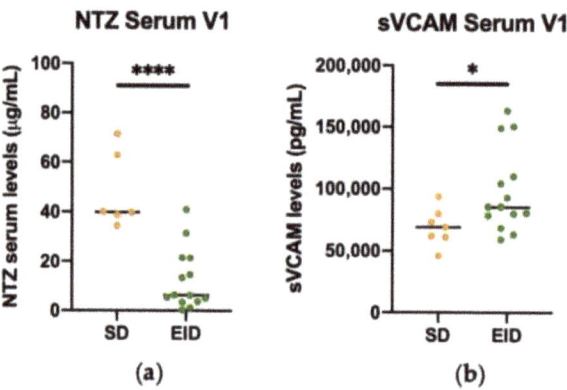

Figure 7. Representation of SD and EID groups in RRMS patients under Natalizumab treatment. Levels of (**a**) NTZ (μg/mL) and (**b**) sVCAM (pg/mL) in serum in the SD ($n = 7$) and EID ($n = 14$) groups. Each dot represents the concentration of NTZ or sVCAM in serum for each patient in the first extraction (V1). EID, extended interval dosing; NTZ, natalizumab; SD, standard dosing; sVCAM, soluble VCAM. ns: $p > 0.05$, * $p < 0.05$, **** $p < 0.0001$.

3.5. Natalizumab Levels in Serum Correlate with CD49d Saturation

The correlation between CD49d saturation levels in CD4$^+$ and CD8$^+$ T lymphocytes and CD19$^+$ lymphocytes and the levels of NTZ and sVCAM in serum was explored. The results showed a positive correlation between CD49d saturation and NTZ in serum for all the lymphocyte subpopulations in both timepoints (Figure 8), while no consistent correlation was observed between CD49d saturation and sVCAM in serum.

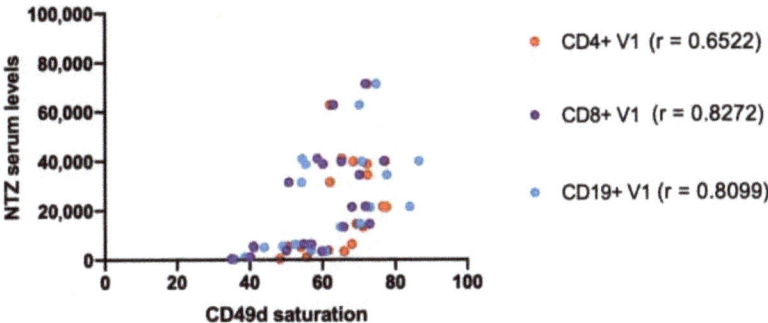

Figure 8. Correlation between Natalizumab serum levels (μg/mL) and CD49d saturation (%) in CD4$^+$ and CD8$^+$ T lymphocytes and CD19$^+$ B lymphocytes in RRMS patients under Natalizumab treatment. Each dot represents a patient of the study (*n* = 29). ns: *p* > 0.05. NTZ: Natalizumab.

4. Discussion and Conclusions

NTZ is one of the most effective treatments for RRMS [20–22], but it has associated a very severe side effect, the risk of developing PML. In this study, we aimed to identify biomarkers to facilitate the development of a personalized dosing regimen for NTZ-treated patients. First, we examined the robustness of several possible cellular and serum biomarkers that could be useful to monitor and personalize NTZ treatment. Here we present data that validates the stability of CD49d saturation and expression as cellular biomarkers in both whole blood and PBMCs as well as the serum protein sVCAM-1. Second, we have explored the impact of an SD schedule and an EID schedule on these markers.

The CNS is an immune-privileged site that generally has sufficient levels of immunosurveillance to protect it against opportunistic infections and neoplastic proliferation. T lymphocytes expressing CD49d play an important role in CNS immunosurveillance. Thus, it has been proposed that CNS immunosurveillance reduction would be the factor that leads to JCV infection in the CNS and PML. One strategy that has been proposed to reduce PML risk is the use of NTZ extended dosing. Previous studies have reported that PML risk was substantially reduced with EID compared to SD, suggesting that the reduction of overall exposure to NTZ can alter PML risk [17]. Nevertheless, little is known about the impact of EID on NTZ pharmacodynamics and pharmacokinetics [19,23]. In this project we aimed to test new biomarkers to monitor NTZ treatment by evaluating the impact of different dosing schedules on NTZ blood levels, the surface expression and saturation of CD49d (as well as their partners CD29 and β7-Integrin).

NTZ binds the CD49d receptor on the surface of leukocytes leading to the saturation of this receptor and changes in its expression. For this reason, the measurement of the saturation and expression levels of CD49d can give information about NTZ binding, which ultimately should impact the effectiveness of the treatment. First, we studied which was the best way to measure such parameters and test if they are stable biomarkers over time to monitor the treatment. To assess the CD49d saturation we performed a protocol previously developed in our lab [19] that consists of a Quantitative Flow Cytometry assay where CD49d and bound NTZ molecules per cell surface are measured to define the saturation of the receptor. The expression of both CD49d and NTZ in whole blood was successfully measured, and it was generally stable over time. Although a few patients showed a large difference in the expression of these parameters between the two timepoints, it could be due to different factors such as intrinsic variability of the patient or the technique. Overall, we consider that CD49d expression measured by this method is very consistent as most of the patients were very stable between V1 and V2. The percentage of saturation of CD49d was also assessed and was also generally found to be quite stable over time and easy to calculate. The instability observed in the CD49d saturation percentage for CD4$^+$ in SD could be explained by the instability in the bound NTZ levels (one of the parameters used to calculate saturation). Moreover, the percentage of CD49d positive cells assessed in PBMCs was also stable overtime. Thus, we demonstrated that CD49d expression and saturation could be assessed by flow cytometry either in whole blood or using PBMCs. Both CD49d saturation and expression were stable within each patient overtime making them potential biomarkers for the clinical practice.

The determination of the saturation levels of CD49d in RRMS patients may allow the definition of a safe saturation range to establish a personalized dose of NTZ for each individual, providing information about whether we must change the dosing schedule or cease NTZ treatment. To this end, we measured and compared the levels of CD49d expression and saturation between SD and EID groups. The results of our study help to describe the pharmacokinetic and pharmacodynamic differences between SD and EID treated patients contributing to better understand how EID impacts on NTZ efficacy and safety. Consistent with previous results obtained in our laboratory [19], we demonstrated that patients receiving SD show a higher percentage (approximately 80%) of CD49d saturation than those in EID (approximately 60%). Interestingly, these higher levels of saturation are not explained by the presence of higher levels of bound NTZ. In fact, both groups showed similar levels of bound NTZ for the studied timepoints, and the difference appears to be due to CD49d expression. Other studies have shown that SD NTZ patients have a decreased expression of CD49d in total PBMCs of approximately 50% and a small (~10%) increase in expression in EID patients [24–26]. Thus, in EID, CD49d expression on the cell-surface should rise as CD49d saturation is reduced indicating a dose-dependent relationship between CD49d surface expression and NTZ serum concentration [19]. In our study, we looked at the specific cell types and could observe significant increases in CD49d expression in CD8$^+$ and CD19$^+$ cells. Although not significant, the number of CD49d molecules on CD4$^+$ cells also appeared higher in EID; we attribute the non-significant result to the sample variation and sample size. When subpopulations of CD8$^+$ and CD19$^+$ cells were assessed, CD49d expression in CD8$^+$ CD27$^+$ and CD19$^+$ DN showed significant increases in the EID group (Figure 4). Taking this into account, we consider CD49d expression as a putative biomarker just in those subpopulations that showed significant differences in both V1 and V2, as they were more consistent. Thus, CD49d expression could be a putative consistent biomarker when analyzing its expression in the previously mentioned CD8$^+$ and CD19$^+$ subpopulations.

The monitoring of CD49d levels allows the identification of patients with different CD49d saturation levels despite being in the same dosing schedule. As performed in this study, NTZ patients can be immunomonitored by Quantitative Flow Cytometry assays to identify patients with suboptimal treatment as well as patients with high levels of saturation that would benefit from EID [19]. The development of news tools for immunomonitoring, such as the one used in this study, contributes to the identification of the optimal NTZ dosing schedule to improve the clinical management and life quality for each RRMS patient. The monitoring and personalization of the treatment could reduce the visits of the patient to the hospital and would allow the patients to achieve proper levels of immunosuppression while maintaining certain levels of immunosurveillance, which could reduce PML risk and other secondary effects of the treatment.

In addition, we checked other parameters in order to search other putative biomarkers that could work as complementary indicators in CD49d monitoring. To do so, we studied the expression of the two beta subunits that form heterodimers with CD49d: CD29 (β1-Integrin) and β7-Integrin. Comparing V1 with V2 suggests that β7-integrin is in general quite stable biomarker over time while CD29 is not, as significant differences were observed between timepoints in several cellular subsets. As we were not able to establish a range of values where they showed significant differences between the two dosing schedule groups, the results suggest that neither CD29 nor β7-Integrin are unlikely to be useful biomarkers to monitor NTZ treatment. This could be probably explained by the fact that these beta subunits also associate with other alpha subunits in T cells to form heterodimers, and we are not detecting just CD49d/CD29 or CD49d/β7-Integrin but also the different heterodimers on cell-surface. Thus, further studies would be needed to determine whether they could be used to monitor NTZ.

Finally, we further studied serum to determine if there was any soluble factor that could be checked to monitor the treatment, since a serum-based biomarker would be much more easily implemented into the clinical practice. The levels of two serum proteins were assessed: NTZ and sVCAM-1. VCAM-1 is an adhesion molecule expressed mainly by in inflamed endothelial cells. It is participating in the firm adhesion of leukocytes to the endothelium, enabling the transmigration of cells into the inflamed tissue [27]. When VLA-4 binds VCAM-1, there is a shedding of the endothelial VCAM-1 that leads to the increase of the concentration of the soluble molecule (sVCAM-1) in serum. The shedding of VCAM-1 from the cell surface and the increase of sVCAM-1 in serum is not specific to the endothelial cerebrovascular cells. However, its increase in patients with MS activity strongly suggests that sVCAM-1 most probably comes from the shedding of VCAM-1 from the activated endothelium of the blood-brain barrier. Because NTZ treatment inhibits leukocyte binding to the endothelium, there is a decrease in sVCAM-1 serum concentration in NTZ treated patients [9,28]. This effect is reversed with the presence of NTZ-neutralizing antibodies in patients, especially when titers are high [28]. Previous studies have suggested a putative role of sVCAM-1 as a sensitive biomarker that could reflect the efficacy of NTZ treatment in MS patients, as its increased concentration in serum is associated with the presence of inflammatory lesions in the CNS [29,30]. As it has been shown that sVCAM-1 serum concentration positively correlates with MS clinical activity [29] and MRI activity [30,31], sVCAM-1 could be a good marker of inflammatory cells binding to the BBB and might serves as a monitoring tool for treatment efficacy. Hence, we studied the sVCAM-1 serum concentrations in SD and EID to test any difference between them that could give indirect information about the BBB cell adhesion. We observed higher levels of sVCAM-1 in blood in EID patients suggesting an increased binding of VLA-4 with its ligand VCAM-1, which may imply an increased trafficking of lymphocytes into the CNS. This could suggest that sVCAM-1 could work as a biomarker to monitor NTZ treatment.

As expected, we observed that patients in SD show higher levels of NTZ in serum than patients in EID, which is in accordance with the administration schedule as patients receiving the treatment more often (4 weeks) have less time to clear NTZ. We observed evident differences in NTZ serum levels between patients which could be explained by differences in how individuals metabolize the drug. Alternatively, this may be the instability observed in the levels of bound NTZ for SD group in the first section (Figure 1b). In brief, our results suggest that both NTZ and sVCAM-1 levels could be used as putative biomarkers to monitor NTZ treatment. To explore the utility of combining serum NTZ levels with other possible biomarkers, a clear correlation between CD49d saturation and NTZ serum levels was observed (Figure 8); this is in agreement with the results obtained by J.Serra López-Matencio et al. [32]. Importantly, since cytometer facilities are not present in all hospitals, monitoring a serum biomarker would be much more feasible to use in routine clinical practice. The positive correlation that we observe between CD49d saturation levels and NTZ levels in serum, suggests that the measurement of NTZ in serum could possibly be used instead of CD49d saturation to monitor the treatment in RRMS patients under NTZ, as was described by Kempen et al. [33]. Hence, it would be very convenient to have a kit to measure NTZ levels in serum to be implemented in the clinical practice.

Regarding the high variability of NTZ levels inside each group, it has been described that the body weight of the patient influences the pharmacodynamic and pharmacokinetic responses to NTZ treatment [19,24]. However, further research is needed to establish pharmacological thresholds of NTZ safety and efficacy, which could help to define the NTZ dosing for each individual patient. Thereby, the variability observed in the studied parameters can be partially explained by factors such as body weight, though different factors could be influencing NTZ metabolism as well [34–36].

In summary, our study shows that CD49d saturation is a stable biomarker that can be used to monitor NTZ-treated RRMS patients, and that could be used to establish a safety range to personalize the treatment. Moreover, the measurement of NTZ levels in serum could be also used in this way in the clinical practice. Finally, further research could also identify sVCAM-1 as a biomarker to achieve the same goal.

Further studies will explore both the cell- and serum-based biomarkers that we have identified with respect NTZ efficacy to assess their potential to develop a personalized dosing schedule for NTZ patients that will maintain efficacy but lower risk of PML.

Author Contributions: Conceptualization, S.G., C.R.-T. and E.M.-C.; methodology, S.G., C.R.-T. and E.M.-C.; software, C.I.-G., A.S.-R. and I.B.; validation, C.I.-G., A.S.-R., A.T.-S. and C.R.-T.; formal analysis, J.G.-G., A.S.-R., S.G., E.M.-C. and C.R.-T.; investigation, J.G.-G., C.I.-G., A.S.-R., S.P.-R., M.J.M., L.B., J.S., M.A.M.-M., E.M., I.B., S.G. and C.R.-T.; resources, S.G., E.M.-C. and C.R.-T.; data curation, C.I.-G., A.S.-R. and A.T.-S.; writing—original draft preparation, J.G.-G.; writing—review and editing, C.I.-G., A.S.-R., A.T.-S., S.P.-R., M.J.M., L.B., J.S., M.A.M.-M., E.M., I.B., S.G., E.M.-C. and C.R.-T.; visualization, J.G.-G.; supervision, S.G., E.M.-C. and C.R.-T.; project administration, E.M.-C. and C.R.-T.; funding acquisition, S.G., E.M.-C. and C.R.-T. All authors have read and agreed to the published version of the manuscript.

Funding: This research was partially sponsored by Biogen Inc. MJM is beneficiary of a Sara Borrell contract from the ISCIII and the FEDER (CD19/00209).

Institutional Review Board Statement: The study was conducted according to the guidelines of the Declaration of Helsinki, and approved by the Ethics Committee of Institut d'Investigació Germans Trias i Pujol (FII-NAT-2015-01, date of approval June 14 2019).

Informed Consent Statement: Informed consent was obtained from all subjects involved in the study.

Acknowledgments: This work has been supported by positive discussion through Consolidated Research Group #2017 SGR 103 (Advanced Immunotherapies for Autoimmunity), AGAUR, Generalitat de Catalunya. The authors are grateful to Katie Whartenby for the critical reading of the manuscript and helpful suggestions. The authors thank Susi Soler for her technical assistance. The authors thank all patients for participating in the study. The authors thank Marco A. Fernández of the Cytometry Facility of IGTP for his continuous help and suggestions.

Conflicts of Interest: S.G. receives compensation from Biogen as a consultant.

Appendix A

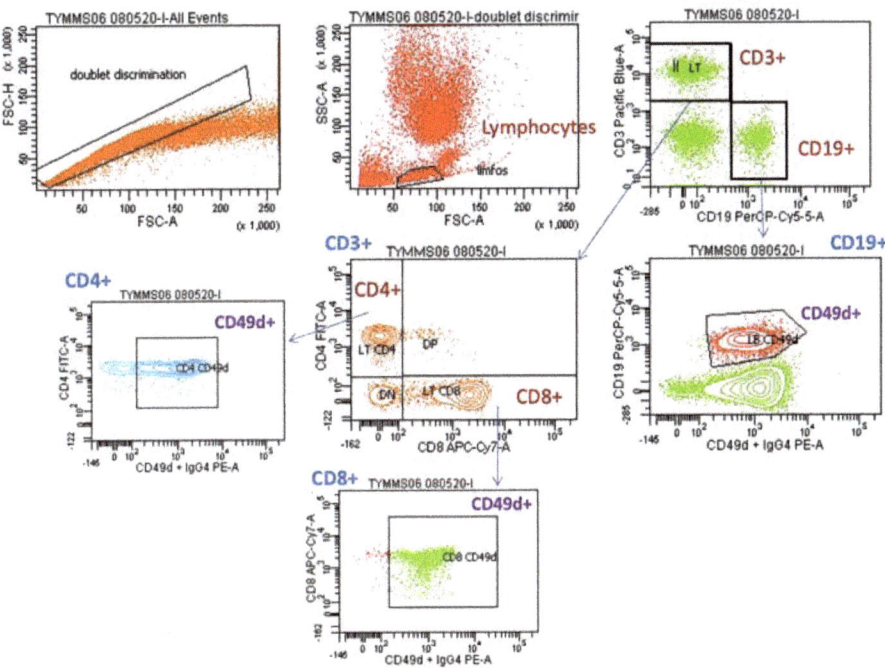

Figure A1. Analysis strategy of the Whole Blood protocol.

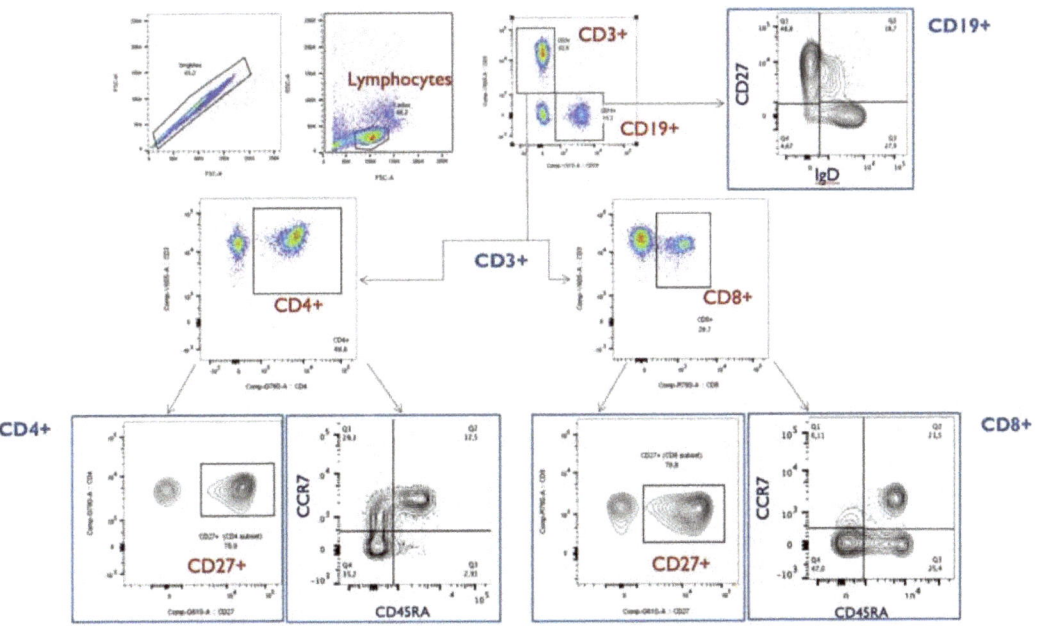

Figure A2. Analysis strategy of the PBMCs protocol.

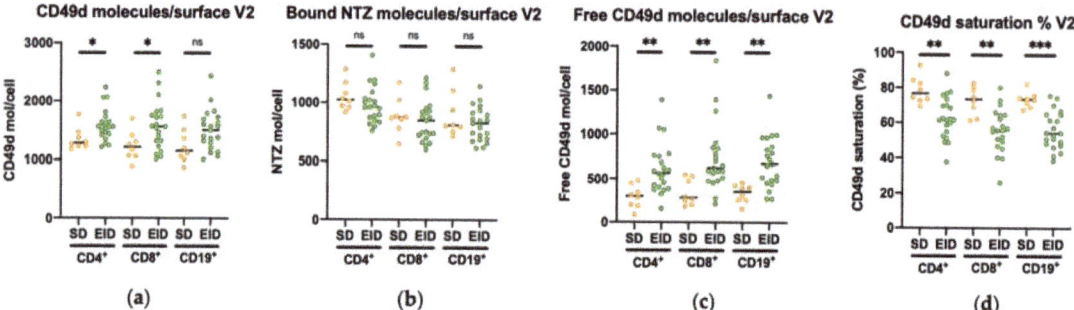

Figure A3. CD49d surface molecules levels and saturation percentage in CD4[+] and CD8[+] T lymphocytes, and CD19[+] B lymphocytes in RRMS patients under Natalizumab treatment in SD or EID. Mean of (**a**) CD49d molecules/cell surface, (**b**) bound NTZ/cell surface, (**c**) free CD49d molecules/cell surface, and (**d**) CD49d saturation percentage in CD4[+] and CD8[+] T lymphocytes, and CD19[+] B lymphocytes in the SD ($n = 8$) and EID ($n = 21$) groups. Each dot represents the number of PE molecules per cell for each patient in the second extraction (V2), translated into the levels of the corresponding antibodies (anti-CD49d PE and huIgG4 Fc PE). EID, extended interval dosing; NTZ, natalizumab; SD, standard dosing. ns: $p > 0.05$, * $p < 0.05$, ** $p < 0.01$, *** $p < 0.001$.

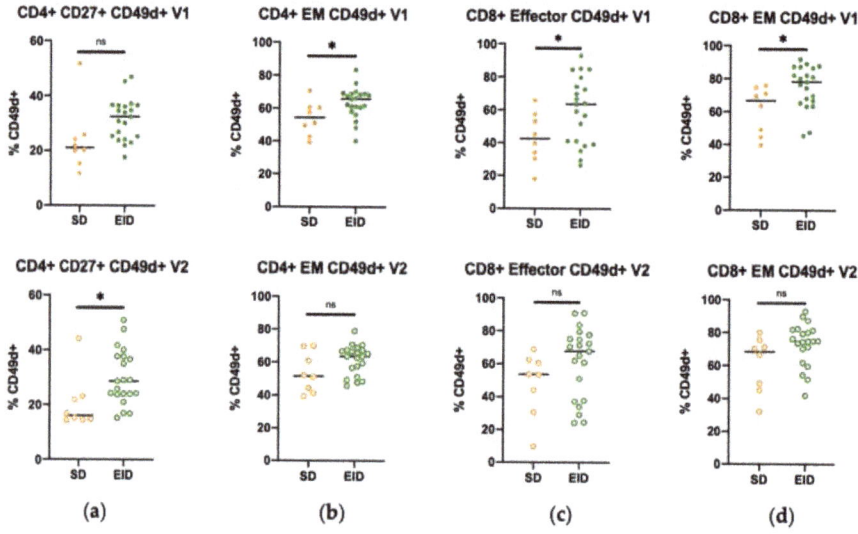

Figure A4. Representation of SD and EID groups in some CD4[+] and CD8[+] T lymphocytes subpopulations in RRMS patients under Natalizumab treatment in both first (V1) and second (V2) extractions. Percentage of expression of CD49d in (**a**) CD4[+]CD27[+], (**b**) CD4[+] Effector Memory (EM), (**c**) CD8[+] Effector and (**d**) CD8[+] Effector Memory (EM) T lymphocytes Each dot represents the percentage of expression for each marker regarding their parent population (CD4[+] or CD8[+] T lymphocytes populations) in the SD ($n = 8$) or EID ($n = 21$) groups. EID, extended interval dosing; EM, effector memory; SD, standard dosing. ns: $p > 0.05$, * $p < 0.05$.

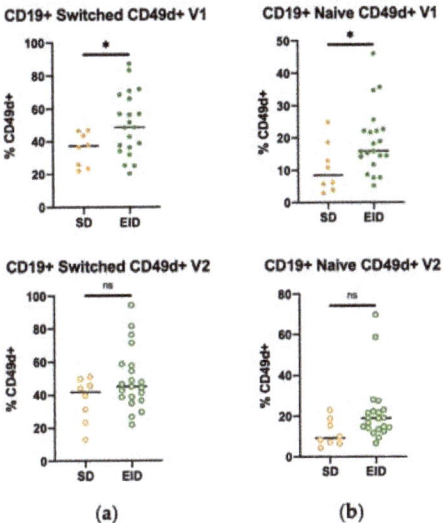

Figure A5. Representation of SD and EID groups in some CD19$^+$ B lymphocytes subpopulations in RRMS patients under Natalizumab treatment in both first (V1) and second (V2) extractions. Percentage of expression of CD49d in (**a**) CD19$^+$ Switched and (**b**) CD19$^+$ Naïve B lymphocytes. Each dot represents the percentage of expression for each marker regarding their parent population (CD19$^+$ B lymphocytes populations) in the SD ($n = 8$) or EID ($n = 21$) groups. EID, extended interval dosing; SD, standard dosing. ns: $p > 0.05$, * $p < 0.05$.

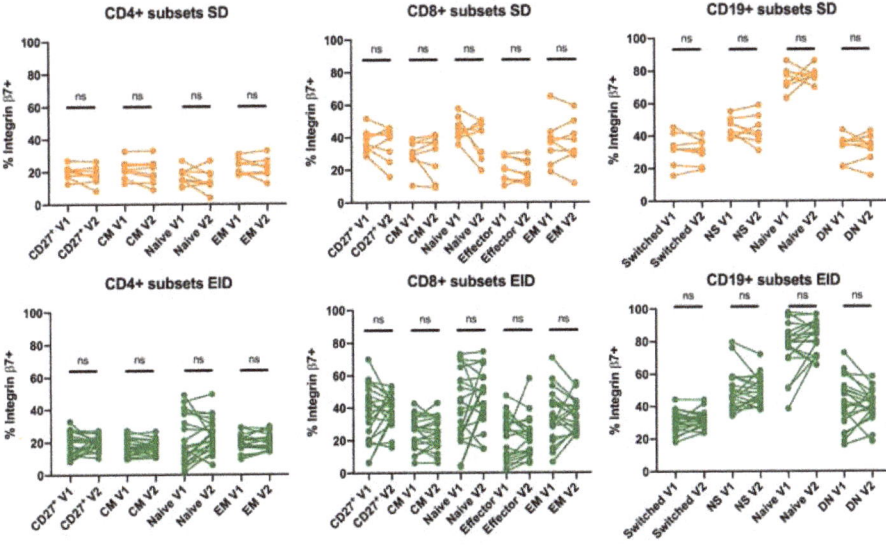

Figure A6. Comparison of first (V1) and second (V2) extractions within CD4$^+$ and CD8$^+$ T lymphocytes, and CD19$^+$ B lymphocytes subpopulations in RRMS patients under Natalizumab treatment in SD or EID. Percentage of expression of β7-Integrin in all CD4$^+$ and CD8$^+$ T lymphocytes, and CD19$^+$ B lymphocytes subsets. Each dot represents the percentage of expression of β7-Integrin regarding their parent population (CD4$^+$ or CD8$^+$ T lymphocytes, or CD19$^+$ B lymphocytes populations) in the SD ($n = 8$) and EID ($n = 21$) groups. CM, Central Memory; DN, Double Negative; EID, extended interval dosing; EM, Effector Memory; NS, Non-Switched; SD, standard dosing. ns: $p > 0.05$.

References

1. Selewski, D.; Shah, G.; Segal, B.; Rajdev, P.; Mukherji, S. Natalizumab (Tysabri). *Am. J. Neuroradiol.* **2010**, *31*, 1588–1590. [CrossRef] [PubMed]
2. Kawamoto, E.; Nakahashi, S.; Okamoto, T.; Imai, H.; Shimaoka, M. Anti-Integrin Therapy for Multiple Sclerosis. *Autoimmune Dis.* **2012**, *2012*, 357101. [CrossRef] [PubMed]
3. Springer, T.A. Traffic signals for lymphocyte recirculation and leukocyte emigration: The multistep paradigm. *Cell* **1994**, *76*, 301–314. [CrossRef]
4. Butcher, E.C. Leukocyte-endothelial cell recognition: Three (or more) steps to specificity and diversity. *Cell* **1991**, *67*, 1033–1036. [CrossRef]
5. Damle, N.K.; Aruffo, A. Vascular cell adhesion molecule 1 induces T-cell antigen receptor-dependent activation of CD4+ T lymphocytes. *Proc. Natl. Acad. Sci. USA* **1991**, *88*, 6403–6407. [CrossRef]
6. Burkly, L.C.; Jakubowski, A.; Newman, B.M.; Rosa, M.D.; Chi-Rosso, G.; Lobb, R.R. Signaling by vascular cell adhesion molecule-1 (VCAM-1) through VLA-4 promotes CD3-dependent T cell proliferation. *Eur. J. Immunol.* **1991**, *21*, 2871–2875. [CrossRef] [PubMed]
7. Wilkins, J.A.; Stupack, D.; Stewart, S.; Caixia, S. β1 Integrin-mediated lymphocyte adherence to extracellular matrix is enhanced by phorbol ester treatment. *Eur. J. Immunol.* **1991**, *21*, 517–522. [CrossRef]
8. Dustin, M.; Springer, T.A. T-cell receptor cross-linking transiently stimulates adhesiveness through LFA-1. *Nature* **1989**, *341*, 619–624. [CrossRef] [PubMed]
9. Petersen, E.; Søndergaard, H.; Oturai, A.; Jensen, P.; Sorensen, P.; Sellebjerg, F.; Börnsen, L. Soluble serum VCAM-1, whole blood mRNA expression and treatment response in natalizumab-treated multiple sclerosis. *Mult. Scler. Relat. Disord.* **2016**, *10*, 66–72. [CrossRef] [PubMed]
10. Brandstadter, R.; Sand, I.K. The use of natalizumab for multiple sclerosis. *Neuropsychiatr. Dis. Treat.* **2017**, *13*, 1691–1702. [CrossRef] [PubMed]
11. Ho, P.-R.; Koendgen, H.; Campbell, N.; Haddock, B.; Richman, S.; Chang, I. Risk of natalizumab-associated progressive multifocal leukoencephalopathy in patients with multiple sclerosis: A retrospective analysis of data from four clinical studies. *Lancet Neurol.* **2017**, *16*, 925–933. [CrossRef]
12. Mancuso, R.; Saresella, M.; Hernis, A.; Marventano, I.; Ricci, C.; Agostini, S.; Rovaris, M.; Caputo, D.; Clerici, M. JC virus detection and JC virus-specific immunity in natalizumab-treated Multiple Sclerosis patients. *J. Transl. Med.* **2012**, *10*, 248. [CrossRef]
13. Ferenczy, M.W.; Marshall, L.J.; Nelson, C.; Atwood, W.J.; Nath, A.; Khalili, K.; Major, E.O. Molecular Biology, Epidemiology, and Pathogenesis of Progressive Multifocal Leukoencephalopathy, the JC Virus-Induced Demyelinating Disease of the Human Brain. *Clin. Microbiol. Rev.* **2012**, *25*, 471–506. [CrossRef] [PubMed]
14. Chesters, P.M.; Heritage, J.; McCance, D.J. Persistence of DNA Sequences of BK Virus and JC Virus in Normal Human Tissues and in Diseased Tissues. *J. Infect. Dis.* **1983**, *147*, 676–684. [CrossRef]
15. Heritage, J.; Chesters, P.M.; McCance, D.J. The persistence of papovavirus BK DNA sequences in normal human renal tissue. *J. Med. Virol.* **1981**, *8*, 143–150. [CrossRef]
16. Rudick, R.A.; Stuart, W.H.; Calabresi, P.A.; Confavreux, C.; Galetta, S.L.; Radue, M.S.E.R.S.E.; Lublin, F.D.; Weinstock-Guttman, B.; Wynn, D.R.; Lynn, F.; et al. Natalizumab plus Interferon Beta-1a for Relapsing Multiple Sclerosis. *N. Engl. J. Med.* **2006**, *354*, 911–923. [CrossRef] [PubMed]
17. Ryerson, L.; Frohman, T.C.; Foley, J.; Kister, I.; Weinstock-Guttman, B.; Tornatore, C.; Pandey, K.; Donnelly, S.; Pawate, S.; Bomprezzi, R.; et al. Extended interval dosing of natalizumab in multiple sclerosis. *J. Neurol. Neurosurg. Psychiatry* **2016**, *87*, 885–889. [CrossRef]
18. European Medicines Agency (EMA). TYSABRI® Product Information. 2009. Available online: https://www.ema.europa.eu/en/documents/product-information/tysabri-epar-product-information_en.pdf (accessed on 2 July 2021).
19. Puñet-Ortiz, J.; Hervás-García, J.V.; Teniente-Serra, A.; Cano-Orgaz, A.; Mansilla, M.J.; Quirant-Sánchez, B.; Navarro-Barriuso, J.; Fernández-Sanmartín, M.A.; Presas-Rodríguez, S.; Ramo-Tello, C.; et al. Monitoring CD49d Receptor Occupancy: A Method to Optimize and Personalize Natalizumab Therapy in Multiple Sclerosis Patients. *Cytom. Part B Clin. Cytom.* **2018**, *94*, 327–333. [CrossRef] [PubMed]
20. Lanzillo, R.; Bonavita, S.; Quarantelli, M.; Vacca, G.; Lus, G.; Amato, L.; Carotenuto, A.; Tedeschi, G.; Orefice, G.; Morra, V.B. Natalizumab is effective in multiple sclerosis patients switching from other disease modifying therapies in clinical practice. *Neurol. Sci.* **2013**, *34*, 521–528. [CrossRef]
21. Butzkueven, H.; Kappos, L.; Pellegrini, F.; Trojano, M.; Wiendl, H.; Patel, R.N.; Zhang, A.; Hotermans, C.; Belachew, S.; on behalf of the TYSABRI Observational Program (TOP) Investigators. Efficacy and safety of natalizumab in multiple sclerosis: Interim observational programme results. *J. Neurol. Neurosurg. Psychiatry* **2014**, *85*, 1190–1197. [CrossRef]
22. Wiendl, H.; Butzkueven, H.; Kappos, L.; Trojano, M.; Pellegrini, F.; Paes, D.; Zhang, A.; Belachew, S. Tysabri® Observational Program (TOP) Investigators Epoch Analysis of On-Treatment Disability Progression Events over Time in the Tysabri Observational Program (TOP). *PLoS ONE* **2016**, *11*, e0144834. [CrossRef]
23. Tanaka, M.; Yokoyama, K. Comparison of nadir serum concentrations in the extended dosing therapy of natalizumab between American and Japanese multiple sclerosis patients. *Mult. Scler. J. Exp. Transl. Clin.* **2016**, *2*. [CrossRef]

24. Foley, J.F.; Goelz, S.; Hoyt, T.; Christensen, A.; Metzger, R.R. Evaluation of natalizumab pharmacokinetics and pharmacodynamics with standard and extended interval dosing. *Mult. Scler. Relat. Disord.* **2019**, *31*, 65–71. [CrossRef]
25. Harrer, A.; Wipfler, P.; Einhaeupl, M.; Pilz, G.; Oppermann, K.; Hitzl, W.; Afazel, S.; Haschke-Becher, E.; Strasser, P.; Trinka, E.; et al. Natalizumab therapy decreases surface expression of both VLA-heterodimer subunits on peripheral blood mononuclear cells. *J. Neuroimmunol.* **2011**, *234*, 148–154. [CrossRef]
26. Sehr, T.; Proschmann, U.; Thomas, K.; Marggraf, M.; Straube, E.; Reichmann, H.; Chan, A.; Ziemssen, T. New insights into the pharmacokinetics and pharmacodynamics of natalizumab treatment for patients with multiple sclerosis, obtained from clinical and in vitro studies. *J. NeuroInflamm.* **2016**, *13*, 164. [CrossRef]
27. Troncoso, M.F.; Ortiz-Quintero, J.; Garrido-Moreno, V.; Sanhueza-Olivares, F.; Guerrero-Moncayo, A.; Chiong, M.; Castro, P.F.; García, L.; Gabrielli, L.; Corbalán, R.; et al. VCAM-1 as a predictor biomarker in cardiovascular disease. *Biochim. Biophys. Acta Mol. Basis Dis.* **2021**, *1867*, 166170. [CrossRef]
28. Millonig, A.; Hegen, H.; Di Pauli, F.; Ehling, R.; Gneiss, C.; Hoelzl, M.; Künz, B.; Lutterotti, A.; Rudzki, D.; Berger, T.; et al. Natalizumab treatment reduces endothelial activity in MS patients. *J. Neuroimmunol.* **2010**, *227*, 190–194. [CrossRef]
29. Hartung, H.-P.; Reiners, K.; Archelos, J.J.; Michels, M.; Seeldrayers, P.; Heidenreich, F.; Pflughaupt, K.W.; Toyka, K.V. Circulating adhesion molecules and tumor necrosis factor receptor in multiple sclerosis: Correlation with magnetic resonance imaging. *Ann. Neurol.* **1995**, *38*, 186–193. [CrossRef] [PubMed]
30. Rieckmann, P.; Altenhofen, B.; Riegel, A.; Felgenhauer, K. Soluble adhesion molecules (sVCAM-1 and sICAM-1) in cerebrospinal fluid and serum correlate with MRI activity in multiple sclerosis. *Ann. Neurol.* **1997**, *41*, 326–333. [CrossRef] [PubMed]
31. Giovannoni, G.; Lai, M.; Thorpe, J.; Kidd, D.; Chamoun, V.; Thompson, A.J.; Miller, D.H.; Feldmann, M. Longitudinal study of soluble adhesion molecules in multiple sclerosis: Correlation with gadolinium enhanced magnetic resonance imaging. *Neurology* **1997**, *48*, 1557–1565. [CrossRef] [PubMed]
32. López-Matencio, J.M.S.; García, Y.P.; Meca-Lallana, V.; Juárez-Sánchez, R.; Ursa, A.; Vega-Piris, L.; Pascual-Salcedo, D.; de Vries, A.; Rispens, T.; Muñoz-Calleja, C. Evaluation of Natalizumab Pharmacokinetics and Pharmacodynamics: Toward Individualized Doses. *Front. Neurol.* **2021**, *12*, 1770. [CrossRef] [PubMed]
33. Van Kempen, Z.L.; Hoogervorst, E.L.; Wattjes, M.P.; Kalkers, N.F.; Mostert, J.P.; Lissenberg-Witte, B.I.; de Vries, A.; Brinke, A.T.; van Oosten, B.W.; Barkhof, F.; et al. Personalized extended interval dosing of natalizumab in MS. *Neurology* **2020**, *95*, e745–e754. [CrossRef] [PubMed]
34. Muralidharan, K.K.; Kuesters, G.; Plavina, T.; Subramanyam, M.; Mikol, D.D.; Gopal, S.; Nestorov, I. Population Pharmacokinetics and Target Engagement of Natalizumab in Patients with Multiple Sclerosis. *J. Clin. Pharmacol.* **2017**, *57*, 1017–1030. [CrossRef]
35. Tanaka, M.; Kinoshita, M.; Foley, J.F.; Tanaka, K.; Kira, J.; Carroll, W.M. Body weight-based natalizumab treatment in adult patients with multiple sclerosis. *J. Neurol.* **2015**, *262*, 781–782. [CrossRef] [PubMed]
36. Biogen. TYSABRI® Prescribing Information. 2004. Available online: https://www.tysabri.com/content/dam/commercial/tysabri/pat/en_us/pdf/tysabri_prescribing_information.pdf (accessed on 25 May 2021).

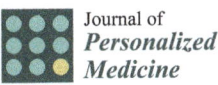

Article

Dynamics and Predictors of Cognitive Impairment along the Disease Course in Multiple Sclerosis

Elisabet Lopez-Soley [1], Eloy Martinez-Heras [1], Magi Andorra [1], Aleix Solanes [2], Joaquim Radua [2,3,4], Carmen Montejo [1], Salut Alba-Arbalat [1], Nuria Sola-Valls [1], Irene Pulido-Valdeolivas [1], Maria Sepulveda [1], Lucia Romero-Pinel [5], Elvira Munteis [6], Jose E. Martínez-Rodríguez [6], Yolanda Blanco [1], Elena H. Martinez-Lapiscina [1], Pablo Villoslada [1], Albert Saiz [1], Elisabeth Solana [1,*,†] and Sara Llufriu [1,*,†]

1. Center of Neuroimmunology, Laboratory of Advanced Imaging in Neuroimmunological Diseases, Hospital Clinic Barcelona, Institut d'Investigacions Biomediques August Pi i Sunyer (IDIBAPS) and Universitat de Barcelona, 08036 Barcelona, Spain; elopez2@clinic.cat (E.L.-S.); emartind@clinic.cat (E.M.-H.); magiandorra@gmail.com (M.A.); c.montejo.gonzalez@gmail.com (C.M.); salba@clinic.cat (S.A.-A.); nuria.sola@grupsagessa.com (N.S.-V.); irenepulidovaldeolivas@gmail.com (I.P.-V.); msepulve@clinic.cat (M.S.); yblanco@clinic.cat (Y.B.); elenahmlapiscina@gmail.com (E.H.M.-L.); pvillos@stanford.edu (P.V.); asaiz@clinic.cat (A.S.)
2. Imaging of Mood- and Anxiety-Related Disorders (IMARD) Group, IDIBAPS and CIBERSAM, 08036 Barcelona, Spain; solanes@clinic.cat (A.S.); radua@clinic.cat (J.R.)
3. Centre for Psychiatry Research, Department of Clinical Neuroscience, Karolinska Institutet, Solna, 171 77 Stockholm, Sweden
4. Early Psychosis: Interventions and Clinical-Detection (EPIC) Laboratory, Department of Psychosis Studies, Institute of Psychiatry, Psychology and Neuroscience, King's College London, London WC2R 2LS, UK
5. Multiple Sclerosis Unit, Neurology Department, Hospital Universitari de Bellvitge, IDIBELL, 08907 Barcelona, Spain; lromeropinel@gmail.com
6. Neurology Department: Hospital del Mar Medical Research Institute (IMIM), 08003 Barcelona, Spain; emunteis@parcdesalutmar.cat (E.M.); jemartinezrguez@gmail.com (J.E.M.-R.)
* Correspondence: elisabeth.solana@idibaps.org (E.S.); sllufriu@clinic.cat (S.L.); Tel.: +34-932275414 (E.S. & S.L.); Fax: +34-932275783 (E.S. & S.L.)
† These authors share co-senior authorship.

Abstract: (1) Background: The evolution and predictors of cognitive impairment (CI) in multiple sclerosis (MS) are poorly understood. We aimed to define the temporal dynamics of cognition throughout the disease course and identify clinical and neuroimaging measures that predict CI. (2) Methods: This paper features a longitudinal study with 212 patients who underwent several cognitive examinations at different time points. Dynamics of cognition were assessed using mixed-effects linear spline models. Machine learning techniques were used to identify which baseline demographic, clinical, and neuroimaging measures best predicted CI. (3) Results: In the first 5 years of MS, we detected an increase in the z-scores of global cognition, verbal memory, and information processing speed, which was followed by a decline in global cognition and memory ($p < 0.05$) between years 5 and 15. From 15 to 30 years of disease onset, cognitive decline continued, affecting global cognition and verbal memory. The baseline measures that best predicted CI were education, disease severity, lesion burden, and hippocampus and anterior cingulate cortex volume. (4) Conclusions: In MS, cognition deteriorates 5 years after disease onset, declining steadily over the next 25 years and more markedly affecting verbal memory. Education, disease severity, lesion burden, and volume of limbic structures predict future CI and may be helpful when identifying at-risk patients.

Keywords: cognition; cognitive impairment; neuroimaging; longitudinal; predictors; multiple sclerosis

1. Introduction

Multiple sclerosis (MS) is a chronic inflammatory demyelinating disease of the central nervous system that entails physical and cognitive impairment (CI). The latter has been reported in 40–70% of people with MS and it has a severe impact on the individual's quality of life [1,2]. CI can be detected in the early phases of MS, but it is more frequent as overall disability accrues [3]. The pattern of cognitive decline predominantly affects information processing speed (IPS) and episodic memory, although executive functions, semantic fluency, and visuospatial analysis may also be altered [4,5]. However, how this deterioration evolves and affects different cognitive domains as the disease progresses is still to be determined.

A few longitudinal studies have investigated the association between clinical and imaging features of MS with cognitive decline, suggesting a predictive value of baseline cognitive status [5], baseline IPS [6], education, and aging [7]. Using different magnetic resonance imaging (MRI) techniques, a relationship has been demonstrated between CI and the combined effect of white matter (WM) and gray matter (GM) damage [8]. In addition, identifying neurodegeneration in specific and cognitively relevant GM regions may help to more accurately predict CI.

Characterizing the natural course of cognitive performance in MS, and identifying predictors of CI, are still distant milestones in clinical MS research. Therefore, in this study, we first describe the temporal dynamics of global cognition and cognitive domains using mixed-effects models, which allowed us to obtain model estimates of specific parameters and to control for between- and within-subject variability. Subsequently, we investigated the baseline demographic, clinical, and MRI measures that best predicted the CI using machine learning (ML) techniques. These issues were addressed in an appropriately large cohort of MS patients with a wide range of disease duration.

2. Materials and Methods

2.1. Participants, Clinical, and Cognitive Assessment

For this longitudinal study, we collected data from a prospective cohort recruited at the MS Unit of the Hospital Clinic of Barcelona from January 2011 to February 2020 [9,10]. The criteria for inclusion in this study were aged between 18 and 65 years, and having at least two clinical and cognitive assessments, with MRI scans available at the first evaluation. Patients did not present any relapse or received any corticosteroid treatment in the last 30 days of the study visit. As such, 212 MS patients fulfilled the inclusion criteria and were analyzed. We collected data regarding sex, age, educational level, disease duration, disease type, the number of relapses before study inclusion, the use of disease-modifying therapies (DMTs), and their global disability evaluated with the Expanded Disability Status Scale (EDSS) [11]. The Ethics Committee at the Hospital Clinic of Barcelona approved the study, and all the participants provided their signed informed consent prior to their enrolment.

At each visit, the participants underwent a neuropsychological evaluation using the Rao's battery [12], with alternate versions when available. Raw values were transformed into z-scores by adjusting for age and education according to the Spanish normative data, and they were grouped in terms of global cognition and for each cognitive domain (verbal and visual memory, attention-IPS, and semantic fluency) [13]. Failure in any test was considered when z-score was below -1.5 standard deviation (SD) of the norm. CI in a given cognitive domain was defined as a failure in at least one test assessing that domain, and global CI was defined as an impairment in at least two cognitive tests evaluating the same or different cognitive domains.

2.2. Magnetic Resonance Imaging (MRI)

2.2.1. MRI Acquisition and Processing

Baseline MRI were acquired on a 3 Tesla Magnetom Trio (SIEMENS, Erlanger, Germany) scanner using a 32-channel phased-array head coil, as described previously [10]. Two different acquisition protocols were used, involving a 3D-Magnetization Prepared Rapid Acquisition Gradient Echo (MPRAGE) and 3D-T2 fluid attenuated inversion recovery (FLAIR) sequence (see Supplementary Material).

2.2.2. Structural MRI Processing for Volumetric Analysis

WM lesions were defined semi-automatically into the 3D-MPRAGE space with the registered 3D-FLAIR image as a reference to improve lesion identification using the Jim7 Software (http://www.xinapse.com/j-im-7-software/). Lesion in-painting was applied to the 3D-MPRAGE image to enhance segmentation and registration. GM regions were parcellated using the Mindboggle software (https://mindboggle.info), applying the Desikan–Killiany Tourville cortical labeling atlas, and the automated subcortical segmentation was achieved with the FSL-FIRST package (fsl.fmrib.ox.ac.uk/fsl/fslwiki/FIRST), resulting in 31 cortical and 7 subcortical labels per hemisphere [14,15]. The volumetric measurements were analyzed using the SIENAX [16] scaling factor to reduce the head-size variability.

We removed interscan variability between the different acquisition protocols using the ComBat function in the R software [17,18].

2.3. Statistical Analysis

All baseline demographic, clinical, and neuroimaging data were described through the median and interquartile range (IQR) or the mean (±SD) for quantitative variables as appropriate as well as through the absolute numbers and the proportions of the qualitative variables. The normal distribution of the data was checked by histograms inspection and using the Shapiro–Wilks test.

We used mixed-effects linear regression to model the dynamics of cognition throughout the course of MS. Models adjusted for age at MS onset, educational level, and sex were used to fit the rates of global cognitive performance and of each cognitive domain using disease duration as a main fixed-effect predictor. In addition, we used linear spline models with the same variables as in the mixed-effects regressions to divide the duration of the disease into three periods. Using visual inspection of the raw data together with prior evidence [19] and the Akaike Information Criterion [20], we selected knots at 5 and 15 years of disease duration to model our data. These models provided three parameters, beta coefficients, for the change in cognition relative to disease duration.

We used ML techniques to identify which baseline demographic, clinical, and MRI measures best serve as predictors of CI. A priori, potential predictor variables were sex, educational level (basic, primary, secondary, or higher), disease duration, disease type, EDSS score, use of DMTs (yes or no), number of relapses before study inclusion, lesion volume, and 76 cortical and subcortical regional volumes [15]. Multiple imputation was employed to handle missing data: we used multiple regression to find the variable distribution and we replaced the missing value by taking a random value from the distribution found. Logistic Lasso regressions were performed to predict the global cognitive status (preserved or impaired, see above). The effect of age was removed from the anatomical brain features, although we included age as a predictor variable in the Lasso model. Lasso regressions automatically select a small number of baseline measures, avoiding overfitting. To validate the performance of the ML models, we used a 10-fold cross-validation method, splitting the overall sample into training and test datasets. We created the imputation algorithms and Lasso regressions using the training datasets alone, while we assessed the performance of the predictions in the independent test datasets. Due to the use of multiple imputation and folds, we created several ML models. We selected the most representative model as the one with the highest overlaps (Dice coefficient) with the other models in the selection of the baseline measures. The same procedure was used for each specific cognitive domain.

All the analyses were performed using the R statistical software (version 3.6.0, www.R-project.org), and the statistical significance was set at $p < 0.05$.

3. Results

A cohort of 212 MS patients who performed a median of three clinical visits per patient (range, 2–5; total assessments = 605) with a median follow-up time of 2.1 years (range 0.9–7.9 years) were included in this study. In terms of the baseline characteristics

(Table 1), the patients were mostly female (68%), middle aged-adults (41 ± 9.47 years), with a relapsing-remitting MS (83%) and with a median disease duration of 8.2 years (range, 0.1–29.0).

Table 1. Demographic, clinical, and MRI characteristics of MS patients at baseline.

	Entire Cohort (n = 212)
Female, n (%)	145 (68)
Age, mean (SD)	41 (9.47)
Educational level, n (%)	
Basic (0–8 years)	16 (8)
Primary (9–12 years)	85 (40)
Secondary (13–16 years)	75 (35)
Higher (>17 years)	36 (17)
Disease duration, median (range)	8.20 (0.1–29.0)
Disease type, n (%)	
Clinically isolated syndrome	19 (9)
Relapsing-remitting MS	176 (83)
Secondary progressive MS	13 (6)
Primary progressive MS	4 (2)
EDSS score, median (range)	2.0 (0–7.0)
Use of DMTs, n (%)	111 (52)
Number of previous relapses, median [IQR]	3 (2–4)
Lesion volume (cm^3), median [IQR]	5.16 (2.37–12.15)

The data represent the absolute numbers and the proportions of the qualitative data, or the median and the interquartile range (IQR) for the quantitative data, unless otherwise specified. SD: standard deviation; MS: multiple sclerosis; EDSS: Expanded Disability Status Scale; DMTs: Disease-Modifying Therapies.

One hundred and eleven patients (52%) were receiving DMTs at baseline, and from them, 94 patients (85%) used moderate-efficacy DMTs (Table S1).

At the latest follow-up, 77 patients (36%) had global CI, 58 patients (27%) had verbal memory impairment, 51 patients (24%) had visual memory impairment, 38 patients (18%) had attention-IPS impairment, and 41 patients (20%) had semantic fluency impairment.

3.1. Cognitive Trajectory throughout Disease Course

According to the linear mixed-effects models, there was an annual cognitive decline that affected verbal memory, visual memory, and semantic fluency (Figure 1A,B, and Table S2). A trend was found in global cognition (p = 0.058), and no significant model was found for attention-IPS (p = 0.345).

When we divided the duration of the disease into three periods, we detected distinct cognitive slopes for each stage (Figure 1C,D and in Table S3). The initial period extended over the first 5 years of the disease, during which an increase in cognition was evident. In the second period, covering 5–15 years of the disease and the third phase, 15–30 years, the cognitive decline in the participants became increasingly accentuated. In the first 5 years of MS, we detected an enhancement in global cognition (β = 0.080 (95% CI, 0.04 to 0.12) z-score/year; p = <0.001), verbal memory (β = 0.083 (95% CI, 0.01 to 0.16) z-score/year; p = 0.037), and attention-IPS (β = 0.107 (95% CI, 0.05 to 0.16) z-score/year; p = <0.001). However, this trajectory was followed by a decline in global cognition (β = −0.029 (95% CI, −0.05 to −0.01) z-score/year; p = 0.013), verbal memory (β = −0.041 (95% CI, −0.08 to 0.00) z-score/year; p = 0.047), and visual memory (β = −0.041 (95% CI, −0.08 to −0.01) z-score/year; p = 0.024) between 5 and 15 years of the disease. Moreover, similar dynamics were observed during the 15–30 years of MS course, during which cognitive decline continued in global cognition (β = −0.031 (95% CI, −0.06 to −0.01) z-score/year; p = 0.021) and verbal memory (β = −0.055 (95% CI, −0.10 to −0.01) z-score/year; emphp = 0.018), and a trend was observed toward a decline in attention-IPS (β = −0.035 (95% CI, −0.07 to 0.00) z-score/year; p = 0.055). No significant effect was detected on semantic fluency performance.

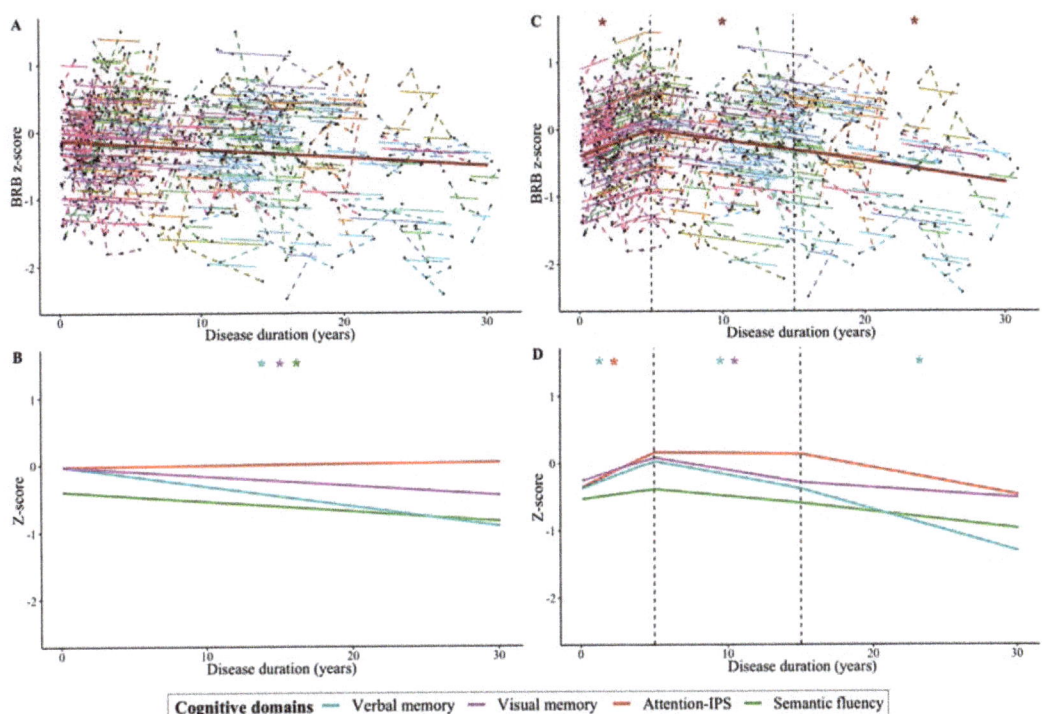

Figure 1. Dynamics of cognitive performance in MS as the disease progresses. The global cognition z-score (**A**) and cognitive domains z-score (**B**) were modeled by mixed-effect regressions. The duration of the disease was divided into three periods by spline models with two knots (at 5 and 15 years of disease duration) represented by dotted black vertical lines (for the global cognition z-score (**C**) and each domain z-score (**D**). Black points joined by a broken line represent the individual trajectories of the changes in the global cognition z-scores, the continuous lines represent the individual fit of the model, and the thicker brown line represents the population model (**A**,**C**). Population model lines of cognitive domains are differentiated by color (**B**,**D**): blue for verbal memory, purple for visual memory, red for attention-IPS, and green for semantic fluency. The x-axis represents the time in years from clinical onset. All models were fitted using the lme4 package in R version 3.5.2 (R Foundation for Statistical Computing: * $p < 0.05$).

3.2. Demographic, Clinical, and MRI Baseline Predictors of Future CI

A Lasso regression was employed to predict CI at the latest follow-up. The models that showed the strongest performance were verbal memory (positive predictive value (PPV) = 62%; negative predictive value (NPV) = 90%) and attention-IPS (PPV = 38%; NPV = 92%), which were more accurate (79% and 73%, respectively) in predicting CI than the other models (Table 2).

The resulting predictive model of global CI included educational level, disease duration, EDSS score, and the number of previous relapses as clinical parameters. The model also included lesion volume and six cortical regional volumes, covering the bilateral parahippocampus, left hippocampus, and right caudate entorhinal and rostral anterior cingulate (Table 3).

Table 2. Performance evaluation of each Lasso regression model.

Cognitive Domain	N	Balanced Accuracy (%)	Sensitivity (%, 95% CI)	Specificity (%, 95% CI)	PPV (%, 95% CI)	NPV (%, 95% CI)
Global cognition	212	71	70 (59–80)	71 (63–79)	58 (47–68)	81 (72–87)
Verbal memory	212	79	76 (63–86)	82 (76–88)	62 (50–73)	90 (84–94)
Visual memory	212	62	71 (56–82)	54 (46–62)	33 (24–42)	85 (77–91)
Attention-IPS	212	73	71 (54–85)	75 (68–81)	38 (27–50)	92 (86–96)
Semantic fluency	210	62	51 (44–59)	73 (57–86)	89 (81–94)	29 (19–36)

Balanced Accuracy is defined as the arithmetic mean of sensitivity and specificity. Sensitivity is defined as the proportion of subjects who developed cognitive impairment that are correctly classified. Specificity is defined as the proportion of subjects who did not develop cognitive impairment that are correctly classified. The predictive model of cognitive impairment in semantic fluency was generated with 210 patients. CI: confidence interval; PPV: positive predictive value; NPV: negative predictive value; IPS: information processing speed.

Table 3. Predictors of each Lasso regression model.

Cognitive Domain	N	Predictors	β	Predictors Selection Rates (Frequency *, %)
Global cognition	212	Educational level	−0.060	1253 (63)
		Disease duration	0.034	936 (47)
		EDSS score	0.325	2000 (100)
		Number of previous relapses	0.069	1635 (82)
		Lesion volume	0.388	2000 (100)
		LH parahippocampal	0.127	1793 (90)
		Left hippocampus	0.070	1595 (80)
		Right caudate	−0.057	1133 (57)
		RH entorhinal	0.044	1087 (54)
		RH parahippocampal	0.085	1836 (92)
		RH rostral anterior cingulate	0.195	1984 (99)
Verbal memory	212	Educational level	−0.386	1983 (99)
		Disease type	0.229	1557 (78)
		EDSS score	0.458	2000 (100)
		Number of previous relapses	0.115	1935 (97)
		Lesion volume	0.309	1998 (100)
		LH parsopercularis	−0.101	1046 (52)
		LH pericalcarine	0.226	1894 (95)
		Left thalamus proper	−0.096	1536 (77)
		Left accumbens area	0.038	1102 (55)
		RH parahippocampal	0.680	2000 (100)
		RH rostral anterior cingulate	0.040	1407 (70)
Visual memory	212	Lesion volume	0.054	1949 (97)
Attention-IPS	212	EDSS score	0.654	2000 (100)
		Lesion volume	0.199	1975 (99)
		LH pericalcarine	0.103	1838 (92)
		Right hippocampus	0.078	0.919 (83)
		RH caudal anterior cingulate	0.035	881 (44)
		RH entorhinal	0.111	1275 (64)
Semantic fluency	210	Lesion volume	−0.019	1005 (50)
		Left hippocampus	−0.017	1071 (53)
		RH rostral anterior cingulate	−0.021	658 (33)

The demographic, clinical, and MRI variables that remained in the age-adjusted predictive model of cognitive impairment in each domain are shown. EDSS: Expanded Disability Status Scale; RH: right hemisphere; LH: left hemisphere; IPS: information processing speed.
* Frequency up to 2000 models.

In terms of verbal memory, CI was predicted by educational level, disease type, EDSS score, and the number of previous relapses. The MRI predictors identified involved lesion volume and six cortical regional volumes, including the right parahippocampus and rostral anterior cingulate, and the pars opercularis, pericalcarine, thalamus, and accumbens of the left hemisphere. Lesion volume was the only predictor selected for CI in terms of visual memory. CI in attention-IPS was predicted by the EDSS, lesion volume and volume of the right hippocampus, caudal anterior cingulate and entorhinal, and the left pericalcarine. The prediction of semantic fluency CI was explained by a model that involved lesion volume and the volume of the left hippocampus and the right rostral anterior cingulate.

4. Discussion

In this longitudinal study, we set out to better understand the deterioration of cognition in MS by describing its temporal dynamics and by identifying predictors of CI. The results reveal different patterns of worsening over the disease course, both in terms of global cognition and the distinct cognitive domains, suggesting a progressive decline after the first 5 years of disease onset that most markedly affects verbal memory. When focusing on the five models that best predicted CI, we found that verbal memory and attention-IPS models had the strongest predictive performance. The results reinforce the importance of the educational level, disease severity, lesion load, and certain GM regional volumes, mainly involving the medial temporal lobe areas and the cingulate, as predictors of cognitive deficits.

There have been some attempts to describe the evolution of cognitive performance in patients with MS, mainly focusing on short time follow-up periods [3,5]. However, the diversity of cohort characteristics and the use of disparate range of cognitive tests and criteria for diagnosing impairment has produced quite heterogeneous data that prove to be difficult to compare across studies. Here, we characterized temporal modifications to different cognitive domains in a cohort of patients with wide ranging disease duration. Our data showed a progressive decline as opposed to an abrupt development of CI, supporting a combined role of age, neurodegeneration, the exhaustion of cognitive reserve, and a loss of plasticity in this clinical manifestation of MS [21]. Moreover, we modeled the trajectory in three different periods by providing differential slopes of the cognitive change during the course of the disease. The results showed an increase in global cognition, verbal memory, and attention-IPS in the first five years after MS onset, which was followed by a decline in cognitive performance. This is a surprising finding even though it is consistent with previous data indicating that cognitive deterioration occurs mainly after the fifth year following disease onset [22]. Several explanations may account for the former. First, it may reflect the capacity of the brain to compensate for the pathological effects of MS lesions through its cognitive reserve, which is a response that may be particularly protective in early stages before structural damage accumulates. Second, the mood disorders such as anxiety or depressive symptoms associated with the diagnosis of MS may negatively affect the results of a first cognitive assessment [23]. Finally, there might be a possible effect of learning in the retesting of cognition that could be present at any stage of the disease, even though we used alternate forms of the tests at each evaluation whenever this was possible.

The cognitive trajectory from the fifth year after MS onset onwards was driven by a decline in verbal and visual memory, although only verbal memory continued to deteriorate until the 30th year of the disease, along with a trend for attention-IPS to decline. Our data reinforce other smaller longitudinal studies, where CI was driven by evolving dysfunction in verbal memory and IPS [5]. By contrast, it was recently shown that IPS was the first domain to be affected [24]. This incongruence may reflect methodological differences, as we grouped the results from the attention-IPS tests into a single cognitive domain, and our cohort also had a lower educational level. Moreover, we cannot rule out a contribution of the distinct cognitive phenotypes in MS [25], as they may differ between cohorts of patients.

Little is known about what may serve to predict the development of CI, hampering research into early prevention and treatment. In the present analysis, the verbal memory and the attention-IPS prediction models produced the highest predictive balanced accuracy and a very high NPV. Educational level was a predictor in the global cognition and verbal memory models, which might reflect the protective role of cognitive reserve in CI [26,27]. In addition, the disease severity indicated by the EDSS and the number of previous relapses seemed to be related to future impairment in global cognition, verbal memory, and attention-IPS models.

Regarding MRI features, global lesion volume was selected as a predictor in all models. In fact, lesion accumulation has been associated with more severe cognitive dysfunction [28] by promoting brain network disruption [10]. Even so, the present results enabled the identification of the specific cortical regional areas related to future cognition. The hippocampus influences global cognition, verbal memory, and semantic fluency, which is consistent with the theory that it is an integral component of the brain network that supports verbal memory and word generation [25,29–31]. Similarly, the volume of the anterior cingulate cortex was present in all predictive models, except for the visual memory model. This region is involved in the fronto-parietal network, and it plays a key role in executive functions, as well as participating in the working memory network [32,33]. Moreover, the thalamus, a highly connected nucleus, has been associated with learning and memory function, and it seems to be a good predictor for CI in MS [5,34], although here, it was more specifically associated with verbal memory impairment. All these areas are part of the limbic system, which plays a crucial role in various cognitive functions [35].

This study has several strengths, including the fact that participants were prospectively and consecutively recruited, thereby preventing a selection bias and enhancing the generalizability of the results. Drawing up a global pattern of cognition in MS was only possible because our cohort included patients with a clinical disease duration of up to 30 years. In addition, all the analyses were performed for global and stratified cognition. Our study also has some limitations. Working with a real-world MS cohort implies that it is predominantly composed of relapsing-remitting MS patients, the most common phenotype encountered clinically in the current treatment era. Moreover, we were unable to assess the influence of mood disorders and fatigue on cognition because, unfortunately, the protocol did not include any mood or fatigue specific test. Furthermore, we do not have a matched control group, although we used z-scores based on normative data to address the changes in cognition that can be expected in accordance with age and educational level. In addition, it has not been possible to analyze the effect of DMTs on cognition, as the predictive models could be influenced by the low proportion of treated patients (52%) at the study initiation predominantly using moderate-efficacy DMTs. Finally, the inclusion of GM lesion volume, WM lesion location, or advanced quantitative MRI measures, such as functional and diffusion MRI, in future studies might be useful to improve our understanding of cognition and its MRI related factors in MS.

5. Conclusions

In conclusion, cognition in MS patients progressively deteriorates after the first 5 years of the disease, with a steady decline over the next 25 years that affects verbal memory more markedly. Moreover, CI is predicted by the educational level, disease severity, lesion load, and volume of high-order regions, including the hippocampus and anterior cingulate cortex, with a strong NPV for the verbal memory and attention-IPS in particular. Consequently, beneficial cognitive maintenance strategies should be adopted that focus on predictors that identify patients at risk of CI and which promote activities such as intellectual enrichment that attenuate the impact of brain burden in the initial years of the disease as an adequate treatment window.

Supplementary Materials: The following are available online at https://www.mdpi.com/article/10.3390/jpm11111107/s1, MRI acquisition parameters, Table S1: Use of disease-modifying therapies at baseline, Table S2: Cognitive changes throughout the disease course, Table S3: Cognitive changes at the different phases of MS.

Author Contributions: Conceptualization, E.L.-S., E.S. and S.L.; Methodology, E.L.-S., E.M.-H., M.A., E.S. and S.L.; Formal Analysis, E.L.-S., M.A., A.S. (Aleix Solanes), J.R. and E.S.; Data Curation, E.L.-S., C.M., S.A.-A., N.S.-V., I.P.-V., M.S., L.R.-P., E.M., J.E.M.-R., Y.B., E.H.M.-L., A.S. (Albert Saiz), E.S. and S.L.; Writing—Original Draft Preparation, E.L.-S., E.M.-H., M.A., A.S. (Aleix Solanes), J.R., E.S. and

S.L.; Writing—Review and Editing, E.L.-S., E.M.-H., M.A., A.S. (Aleix Solanes), J.R., E.S. and S.L.; Supervision, E.H.M.-L., P.V., A.S. (Albert Saiz), E.S. and S.L.; Project Administration, A.S. (Albert Saiz) and S.L.; Funding Acquisition, A.S. (Albert Saiz) and S.L. All authors have read and agreed to the published version of the manuscript.

Funding: The author(s) disclose receipt of the following financial support for the research, authorship, and/or publication of this article. This work was funded by: a Proyecto de Investigación en Salud (PI15/00587 to S.LL., and A.S.; PI15/00061 to P.V.; PI18/01030 to S.LL. and A.S.; and JR16/00006; MV17/00021; PI17/01228; RD16/0015/0003 to E.H.M-L.), integrated into the Plan Estatal de Investigación Científica y Técnica de Innovación I+D+I, and co-funded by the Instituto de Salud Carlos III-Subdirección General de Evaluación and the Fondo Europeo de Desarrollo Regional (FEDER, "Otra manera de hacer Europa"); by the Red Española de Esclerosis Múltiple (REEM: RD16/0015/0002, RD16/0015/0003, RD12/0032/0002, RD12/0060/01-02); by TEVA Spain, the Ayudas Merck de Investigación 2017 from the Fundación Merck Salud and the Proyecto Societat Catalana Neurologia 2017; and by the MS Innovation GMSI, 2016 to E.H.M.-L., E.L.-S. holds a predoctoral grant from the University of Barcelona (APIF). M.A. holds equities in Bionure and Goodgut. C.M. was awarded by the Hospital Clinic Emili Letang, and she holds a P-FIS contract (FI19/00111). J.R. holds a Miguel Servet Research Contract (CPII19/00009) and Research Project PI19/00394 from the Plan Nacional de I+D+I 2013–2016, the Instituto de Salud Carlos III-Subdirección General de Evaluación y Fomento de la Investigación and the European Regional Development Fund (FEDER, 'Investing in your future'). None of the funding bodies had any role in the design and performance of the study; the collection, management, analysis, and interpretation of the data; the preparation, revision, or approval of the manuscript; and the decision to submit the manuscript for publication.

Institutional Review Board Statement: The study was conducted according to the guidelines of the Declaration of Helsinki and approved by the Ethics Committee of the Hospital Clinic of Barcelona (protocol code HCB/2009/4905 on 7 April 2009; protocol code HCB/2015/0236 on 23 November 2015; protocol code HCB/2912/7965 on 2 December 2015; protocol code HCB/2016/0827 on 12 December 2016).

Informed Consent Statement: Informed consent was obtained from all subjects involved in the study.

Data Availability Statement: The datasets generated during and/or analyzed in the current study are available from the corresponding authors upon reasonable request.

Acknowledgments: The authors are grateful to Núria Bargalló, Cesar Garrido and the IDIBAPS Magnetic resonance imaging facilities, and to the Fundació Cellex for their support of this study. This work was carried out at the Centro Esther Koplowitz of the IDIBAPS (Barcelona, Spain), which is supported by the CERCA Programme/Generalitat de Catalunya.

Conflicts of Interest: The authors declare the following potential conflicts of interest with respect to their research, authorship, and/or the publication of this article: E.M.-H., A.S., J.R., C.M. and S.A.-A. have nothing to disclose; E.L.-S. and E.S. received travel reimbursement from Sanofi and ECTRIMS; M.A. holds equity shares of Bionure, S.L. and Goodgut S.L., stock options for Attune Neurosciences Inc., and he is currently an employee of Roche, although his contribution to this work is associated with his previous work at IDIBAPS; N.S.-V. received compensation for consulting services and speaker honoraria from Genzyme-Sanofi, Almirall, Novartis, Roche and Almirall; I.P.-V. received travel reimbursement from Roche and Genzyme, she holds stock options in Aura Innovative Robotics and currently, she is an employee at UCB Pharma, the contribution to this study is associated with her previous work at IDIBAPS; M.S. received speaker honoraria from Genzyme, Novartis, and Biogen; L.R.-P. received honoraria compensation to participate in advisory boards, collaborations as a consultant and scientific communications and received research support, funding for travel, and congress expenses from Biogen Idec, Novartis, TEVA, MerckSerono, Genzyme, Almirall, Bayer, Celgene and Roche; E.M. received speaking honoraria from Merck and Novartis; J.E.M.-R. has participated as principal investigators in pharmaceutical company-sponsored clinical trials by Novartis, Roche, Merck-Serono, Actelion, Celgene, Oryzon Genomics, and Medday, carried out at the Hospital del Mar, IMIM, Barcelona. J.E.M.-R. also received fees for consulting services and lectures from Novartis, Sanofi and Biogen Idec, and travel funding from Biogen Idec and Sanofi; Y.B. received speaking honoraria from Biogen, Novartis, and Genzyme; E.H.M.-L. received travel support for international and national meetings from Roche and Sanofi-Genzyme, and honoraria for consultancies from Novartis, Roche, and Sanofi before joining the European Medicines Agency where she is currently employed (Human Medicines, since 16 April 2019), although her contribution to this article is related to her activity at the Hospital Clinic of Barcelona/IDIBAPS and consequently, it does not represent the views of the Agency or its Committees. She is a member of the International Multiple Sclerosis Visual System (IMSVISUAL) Consortium; P.V. is a shareholder and has received consultancy fees from Accure Therapeutics SL, Attunne Neurosciences Inc., QMenta Inc., Spiral Therapeutix Inc, CLight Inc. and NeuroPrex Inc., as well as having held grants from the Instituto de Salud Carlos III and the European Commissions; A.S. received compensation for consulting services and speaker honoraria from Bayer-Schering, Merck-Serono, Biogen-Idec, Sanofi-Aventis, TEVA, Novartis and Roche; S.L. received compensation for consulting services and speaker honoraria from Biogen Idec, Novartis, TEVA, Genzyme, Sanofi and Merck.

References

1. Chiaravalloti, N.D.; DeLuca, J. Cognitive Impairment in Multiple Sclerosis. *Lancet Neurol.* **2008**, *7*, 1139–1151. [CrossRef]
2. Højsgaard Chow, H.; Schreiber, K.; Magyari, M.; Ammitzbøll, C.; Börnsen, L.; Romme Christensen, J.; Ratzer, R.; Soelberg Sørensen, P.; Sellebjerg, F. Progressive Multiple Sclerosis, Cognitive Function, and Quality of Life. *Brain Behav.* **2018**, *8*, e00875. [CrossRef] [PubMed]
3. Amato, M.P.; Portaccio, E.; Goretti, B.; Zipoli, V.; Hakiki, B.; Giannini, M.; Pastò, L.; Razzolini, L. Cognitive Impairment in Early Stages of Multiple Sclerosis. *Neurol. Sci.* **2010**, *31*, 211–214. [CrossRef] [PubMed]
4. Sumowski, J.F.; Benedict, R.; Enzinger, C.; Filippi, M.; Geurts, J.J.; Hamalainen, P.; Hulst, H.; Inglese, M.; Leavitt, V.M.; Rocca, M.A.; et al. Cognition in Multiple Sclerosis: State of the Field and Priorities for the Future. *Neurology* **2018**, *90*, 278–288. [CrossRef]
5. Damasceno, A.; Pimentel-Silva, L.R.; Damasceno, B.P.; Cendes, F. Cognitive Trajectories in Relapsing–remitting Multiple Sclerosis: A Longitudinal 6-Year Study. *Mult. Scler.* **2020**, *26*, 1740–1751. [CrossRef]
6. Heled, E.; Aloni, R.; Achiron, A. Cognitive Functions and Disability Progression in Relapsing-Remitting Multiple Sclerosis: A Longitudinal Study. *Appl. Neuropsychol. Adult* **2021**, *28*, 210–219. [CrossRef]
7. Eijlers, A.J.C.; Meijer, K.A.; van Geest, Q.; Geurts, J.J.G.; Schoonheim, M.M. Determinants of Cognitive Impairment in Patients with Multiple Sclerosis with and without Atrophy. *Radiology* **2018**, *288*, 544–551. [CrossRef]
8. Di Filippo, M.; Portaccio, E.; Mancini, A.; Calabresi, P. Multiple Sclerosis and Cognition: Synaptic Failure and Network Dysfunction. *Nat. Rev. Neurosci.* **2018**, *19*, 599–609. [CrossRef]
9. Martínez-Lapiscina, E.H.; Fraga-Pumar, E.; Gabilondo, I.; Martínez-Heras, E.; Torres-Torres, R.; Ortiz-Pérez, S.; Llufriu, S.; Tercero, A.; Andorra, M.; Roca, M.F.; et al. The Multiple Sclerosis Visual Pathway Cohort: Understanding Neurodegeneration in MS. *BMC Res. Notes* **2014**, *7*, 910. [CrossRef] [PubMed]
10. Llufriu, S.; Martinez-Heras, E.; Solana, E.; Sola-Valls, N.; Sepulveda, M.; Blanco, Y.; Martinez-Lapiscina, E.H.; Andorra, M.; Villoslada, P.; Prats-Galino, A.; et al. Structural Networks Involved in Attention and Executive Functions in Multiple Sclerosis. *NeuroImage Clin.* **2017**, *13*, 288–296. [CrossRef] [PubMed]
11. Kurtzke, J.F. Rating Neurologic Impairment in Multiple Sclerosis: An Expanded Disability Status Scale (EDSS). *Neurology* **1983**, *33*, 1444–1452. [CrossRef]
12. Rao, S.M.; Leo, G.J.; Bernardin, L.; Unverzagt, F. Cognitive Dysfunction in Multiple Sclerosis. I. Frequency, Patterns, and Prediction. *Neurology* **1991**, *41*, 685–691. [CrossRef] [PubMed]
13. Sepulcre, J.; Vanotti, S.; Hernández, R.; Sandoval, G.; Cáceres, F.; Garcea, O.; Villoslada, P. Cognitive Impairment in Patients with Multiple Sclerosis Using the Brief Repeatable Battery-Neuropsychology Test. *Mult. Scler.* **2006**, *12*, 187–195. [CrossRef]
14. Klein, A.; Ghosh, S.S.; Bao, F.S.; Giard, J.; Häme, Y.; Stavsky, E.; Lee, N.; Rossa, B.; Reuter, M.; Chaibub Neto, E.; et al. Mindboggling Morphometry of Human Brains. *PLoS Comput. Biol.* **2017**, *13*, e1005350. [CrossRef] [PubMed]
15. Desikan, R.S.; Ségonne, F.; Fischl, B.; Quinn, B.T.; Dickerson, B.C.; Blacker, D.; Buckner, R.L.; Dale, A.M.; Maguire, R.P.; Hyman, B.T.; et al. An Automated Labeling System for Subdividing the Human Cerebral Cortex on MRI Scans into Gyral Based Regions of Interest. *Neuroimage* **2006**, *31*, 968–980. [CrossRef]
16. Smith, S.M.; Jenkinson, M.; Woolrich, M.W.; Beckmann, C.F.; Behrens, T.E.J.; Johansen-Berg, H.; Bannister, P.R.; De Luca, M.; Drobnjak, I.; Flitney, D.E.; et al. Advances in Functional and Structural MR Image Analysis and Implementation as FSL. *Neuroimage* **2004**, *23* (Suppl. S1), S208–S219. [CrossRef]
17. Fortin, J.-P.; Parker, D.; Tunç, B.; Watanabe, T.; Elliott, M.A.; Ruparel, K.; Roalf, D.R.; Satterthwaite, T.D.; Gur, R.C.; Gur, R.E.; et al. Harmonization of Multi-Site Diffusion Tensor Imaging Data. *Neuroimage* **2017**, *161*, 149–170. [CrossRef] [PubMed]
18. Radua, J.; Vieta, E.; Shinohara, R.; Kochunov, P.; Quidé, Y.; Green, M.J.; Weickert, C.S.; Weickert, T.; Bruggemann, J.; Kircher, T.; et al. Increased Power by Harmonizing Structural MRI Site Differences with the ComBat Batch Adjustment Method in ENIGMA. *Neuroimage* **2020**, *218*, 116956. [CrossRef]
19. Scalfari, A.; Neuhaus, A.; Daumer, M.; Muraro, P.A.; Ebers, G.C. Onset of Secondary Progressive Phase and Long-Term Evolution of Multiple Sclerosis. *J. Neurol. Neurosurg. Psychiatry* **2014**, *85*, 67–75. [CrossRef]
20. Akaike, H. A New Look at the Statistical Model Identification. *Springer Ser. Stat.* **1974**, 215–222.
21. Mahad, D.H.; Trapp, B.D.; Lassmann, H. Pathological Mechanisms in Progressive Multiple Sclerosis. *Lancet Neurol.* **2015**, *14*, 183–193. [CrossRef]

22. Achiron, A.; Chapman, J.; Magalashvili, D.; Dolev, M.; Lavie, M.; Bercovich, E.; Polliack, M.; Doniger, G.M.; Stern, Y.; Khilkevich, O.; et al. Modeling of Cognitive Impairment by Disease Duration in Multiple Sclerosis: A Cross-Sectional Study. *PLoS ONE* **2013**, *8*, e71058.
23. Leavitt, V.M.; Brandstadter, R.; Fabian, M.; Sand, I.K.; Klineova, S.; Krieger, S.; Lewis, C.; Lublin, F.; Miller, A.; Pelle, G.; et al. Dissociable Cognitive Patterns Related to Depression and Anxiety in Multiple Sclerosis. *Mult. Scler. J.* **2020**, *26*, 1247–1255. [CrossRef]
24. Wojcik, C.; Fuchs, T.A.; Tran, H.; Dwyer, M.G.; Jakimovski, D.; Unverdi, M.; Weinstock-Guttman, B.; Zivadinov, R.; Eshaghi, A.; Benedict, R.H. Staging and Stratifying Cognitive Dysfunction in Multiple Sclerosis. *Mult. Scler.* **2021**, 13524585211011390.
25. De Meo, E.; Portaccio, E.; Giorgio, A.; Ruano, L.; Goretti, B.; Niccolai, C.; Patti, F.; Chisari, C.G.; Gallo, P.; Grossi, P.; et al. Identifying the Distinct Cognitive Phenotypes in Multiple Sclerosis. *JAMA Neurol.* **2021**, *78*, 414–425. [CrossRef]
26. Sumowski, J.F.; Chiaravalloti, N.; DeLuca, J. Cognitive Reserve Protects against Cognitive Dysfunction in Multiple Sclerosis. *J. Clin. Exp. Neuropsychol.* **2009**, *31*, 913–926. [CrossRef] [PubMed]
27. Lopez-Soley, E.; Solana, E.; Martínez-Heras, E.; Andorra, M.; Radua, J.; Prats-Uribe, A.; Montejo, C.; Sola-Valls, N.; Sepulveda, M.; Pulido-Valdeolivas, I.; et al. Impact of Cognitive Reserve and Structural Connectivity on Cognitive Performance in Multiple Sclerosis. *Front. Neurol.* **2020**, *11*, 581700. [CrossRef] [PubMed]
28. Papadopoulou, A.; Müller-Lenke, N.; Naegelin, Y.; Kalt, G.; Bendfeldt, K.; Kuster, P.; Stoecklin, M.; Gass, A.; Sprenger, T.; Radue, E.W.; et al. Contribution of Cortical and White Matter Lesions to Cognitive Impairment in Multiple Sclerosis. *Mult. Scler.* **2013**, *19*, 1290–1296. [CrossRef]
29. Glikmann-Johnston, Y.; Oren, N.; Hendler, T.; Shapira-Lichter, I. Distinct Functional Connectivity of the Hippocampus during Semantic and Phonemic Fluency. *Neuropsychologia* **2015**, *69*, 39–49. [CrossRef] [PubMed]
30. Llufriu, S.; Rocca, M.A.; Pagani, E.; Riccitelli, G.C.; Solana, E.; Colombo, B.; Rodegher, M.; Falini, A.; Comi, G.; Filippi, M. Hippocampal-Related Memory Network in Multiple Sclerosis: A Structural Connectivity Analysis. *Mult. Scler.* **2019**, *25*, 801–810. [CrossRef]
31. Sepulcre, J.; Masdeu, J.C.; Sastre-Garriga, J.; Goñi, J.; Vélez-de-Mendizábal, N.; Duque, B.; Pastor, M.A.; Bejarano, B.; Villoslada, P. Mapping the Brain Pathways of Declarative Verbal Memory: Evidence from White Matter Lesions in the Living Human Brain. *Neuroimage* **2008**, *42*, 1237–1243. [CrossRef] [PubMed]
32. Weygandt, M.; Wakonig, K.; Behrens, J.; Meyer-Arndt, L.; Söder, E.; Brandt, A.U.; Bellmann-Strobl, J.; Ruprecht, K.; Gold, S.M.; Haynes, J.-D.; et al. Brain Activity, Regional Gray Matter Loss, and Decision-Making in Multiple Sclerosis. *Mult. Scler.* **2018**, *24*, 1163–1173. [CrossRef] [PubMed]
33. Sepulcre, J.; Masdeu, J.C.; Pastor, M.A.; Goñi, J.; Barbosa, C.; Bejarano, B.; Villoslada, P. Brain Pathways of Verbal Working Memory: A Lesion-Function Correlation Study. *Neuroimage* **2009**, *47*, 773–778. [CrossRef] [PubMed]
34. Amin, M.; Ontaneda, D. Thalamic Injury and Cognition in Multiple Sclerosis. *Front. Neurol.* **2020**, *11*, 623914. [CrossRef]
35. Keser, Z.; Hasan, K.M.; Mwangi, B.; Younes, K.; Khayat-Khoei, M.; Kamali, A.; Lincoln, J.A.; Nelson, F.M. Quantitative Limbic System Mapping of Main Cognitive Domains in Multiple Sclerosis. *Front. Neurol.* **2018**, *9*, 132. [CrossRef]

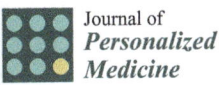

Journal of Personalized Medicine

Article

Cognitive Performance and Health-Related Quality of Life in Patients with Neuromyelitis Optica Spectrum Disorder

Elisabet Lopez-Soley [1,†], Jose E. Meca-Lallana [2,†], Sara Llufriu [1], Yolanda Blanco [1], Rocío Gómez-Ballesteros [3], Jorge Maurino [3], Francisco Pérez-Miralles [4], Lucía Forero [5], Carmen Calles [6], María L. Martinez-Gines [7], Inés Gonzalez-Suarez [8], Sabas Boyero [9], Lucía Romero-Pinel [10], Ángel P. Sempere [11], Virginia Meca-Lallana [12], Luis Querol [13], Lucienne Costa-Frossard [14], Maria Sepulveda [1,‡] and Elisabeth Solana [1,*,‡]

1. Center of Neuroimmunology, Laboratory of Advanced Imaging in Neuroimmunological Diseases, Hospital Clinic Barcelona, Institut d'Investigacions Biomediques August Pi i Sunyer (IDIBAPS) and Universitat de Barcelona, 08036 Barcelona, Spain; elopez2@clinic.cat (E.L.-S.); sllufriu@clinic.cat (S.L.); yblanco@clinic.cat (Y.B.); msepulve@clinic.cat (M.S.)
2. Department of Neurology, Clinical Neuroimmunology Unit and Multiple Sclerosis CSUR, Hospital Universitario "Virgen de la Arrixaca", IMIB-Arrixaca, 30120 Murcia, Spain; pmecal@gmail.com
3. Medical Department, Roche Farma, 28042 Madrid, Spain; rocio.gomez@roche.com (R.G.-B.); jorge.maurino@roche.com (J.M.)
4. Department of Neurology, Unit of Neuroimmunology, Hospital Universitari i Politècnic La Fe, 46026 Valencia, Spain; miralles_neuro@hotmail.com
5. Department of Neurology, Hospital Universitario Puerta del Mar, 11009 Cadiz, Spain; lucia.forero.diaz@hotmail.com
6. Department of Neurology, Hospital Universitari Son Espases, 07120 Palma de Mallorca, Spain; mcalles22@yahoo.es
7. Department of Neurology, Hospital Universitario Gregorio Marañón, 28007 Madrid, Spain; marisamgines@hotmail.com
8. Department of Neurology, Hospital Universitario Álvaro Cunqueiro, 36213 Vigo, Spain; igonsua@gmail.com
9. Department of Neurology, Hospital Universitario Cruces, 48903 Bilbao, Spain; sabasboyero@gmail.com
10. Department of Neurology, Hospital Universitari de Bellvitge, 08907 Barcelona, Spain; lromeropinel@gmail.com
11. Department of Neurology, Hospital General Universitario de Alicante, 03010 Alicante, Spain; aperezs@mac.com
12. Department of Neurology, Hospital Universitario La Princesa, 28006 Madrid, Spain; virmeca@hotmail.com
13. Department of Neurology, Hospital de la Santa Creu i Sant Pau, 08025 Barcelona, Spain; lquerol@santpau.cat
14. Department of Neurology, Hospital Universitario Ramón y Cajal, 28034 Madrid, Spain; lufrossard@yahoo.es
* Correspondence: elisabeth.solana@idibaps.org
† These authors contributed equally to this work and share first authorship.
‡ These authors contributed equally to this work and share co-senior authorship.

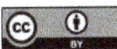

Abstract: Background: The frequency of cognitive impairment (CI) reported in neuromyelitis optica spectrum disorder (NMOSD) is highly variable, and its relationship with demographic and clinical characteristics is poorly understood. We aimed to describe the cognitive profile of NMOSD patients, and to analyse the cognitive differences according to their serostatus; furthermore, we aimed to assess the relationship between cognition, demographic and clinical characteristics, and other aspects linked to health-related quality of life (HRQoL). Methods: This cross-sectional study included 41 patients (median age, 44 years; 85% women) from 13 Spanish centres. Demographic and clinical characteristics were collected along with a cognitive z-score (Rao's Battery) and HRQoL patient-centred measures, and their relationship was explored using linear regression. We used the Akaike information criterion to model which characteristics were associated with cognition. Results: Fourteen patients (34%) had CI, and the most affected cognitive domain was visual memory. Cognition was similar in AQP4-IgG-positive and -negative patients. Gender, mood, fatigue, satisfaction with life, and perception of stigma were associated with cognitive performance (adjusted $R^2 = 0.396$, $p < 0.001$). Conclusions: The results highlight the presence of CI and its impact on HRQoL in NMOSD patients. Cognitive and psychological assessments may be crucial to achieve a holistic approach in patient care.

Keywords: neuromyelitis optica spectrum disorder; cognition; health-related quality of life; mood

1. Introduction

Neuromyelitis optica spectrum disorder (NMOSD) is an inflammatory autoimmune disorder of the central nervous system (CNS) predominantly targeting the spinal cord and optic nerve [1,2]. The discovery of an immunoglobulin G directed against the astrocyte water channel protein aquaporin-4 (AQP4-IgG) not only allowed a reliable distinction of the disease from multiple sclerosis (MS), the most common differential diagnosis [3], but also led to expansion of the clinical syndromes associated with the disorder and the definition of a new set of diagnostic criteria with prognostic implications (2015 criteria) [4].

Most NMOSD patients follow a course of early disability accrual due to frequent and potentially severe relapses. In recent years, increasing attention has been paid to the prevalence and pattern of cognitive impairment (CI) in NMOSD patients, as it is an underestimated but disabling symptom with imprecise description [5]. The frequency of CI varies substantially across studies, ranging from 3% to 75% [6,7], with methodological heterogeneity in terms of samples enrolled, diagnostic criteria applied, CI definition or the neuropsychological assessment tools employed [1,7,8]. Previous studies not only have high variations across the frequency of CI, but also depict ambiguous results about the most affected cognitive domains in NMOSD patients. Moreover, it is not entirely clear whether the presence or absence of AQP4-IgG could influence cognitive performance.

Other aspects related to the disease, such as mood, fatigue, and self-perception of symptoms and pain have an impact on the patient's quality of life, interfering with physical and emotional aspects of wellbeing [9,10]. However, the relationship of these factors with NMOSD patients' cognitive performance has been poorly investigated. A further analysis of the full spectrum of cognitive performance and the impact of psychological comorbidities is needed for a better understanding of the disease's symptoms, and to provide potential target interventions. Therefore, the main objective of this study was to describe the cognitive profile of a well-characterised group of patients with NMOSD, and to analyse cognitive differences according to their serostatus. The secondary objective was to assess the relationship between cognition, demographic and clinical characteristics, and the contribution of emotional status and other aspects related to the health-related quality of life (HRQoL).

2. Materials and Methods

2.1. Participants

For this non-interventional cross-sectional study, we collected data from patients consecutively recruited at thirteen hospital-based neuroimmunology clinics in Spain (PERSPECTIVES-NMO study) [11] between November 2019 and July 2020. The inclusion criteria were (a) patients aged between 18 and 65 years; (b) diagnosed with NMOSD according to the Wingerchuk 2015 criteria [4]; (c) relapse-free or not having received corticosteroids in the last 30 days; (d) stable treatment in the last three months and; (e) available cognitive and mood disorder assessments. Patients with difficulties in understanding and/or responding to the study questionnaires and with other concomitant chronic disorders that could significantly affect cognition or mood were excluded from the study.

Thus, a total of 41 NMOSD patients fulfilled the inclusion criteria and were analysed. Epidemiological and clinical data (age, gender, educational level, disease duration, presence of AQP4-IgG antibodies, number of relapses, and current treatment) were recorded in an electronic case report form specially designed for this study. Neurological disability was assessed by the Expanded Disability Status Scale (EDSS) score [12]. We evaluated mood disorders using the Beck Depression Inventory-Fast Screen (BDI-FS) [13], with a total score ranging from 0 to 21. Higher scores indicate more severe depression symptoms with cut-off scores ≥ 4, ≥ 9, and >12 indicating mild, moderate, and severe depression, respectively.

Daily fatigue was assessed by the Fatigue Impact Scale for Daily Use (D-FIS) [14], an 8-item self-report instrument in which higher scores indicate a greater impact of fatigue. The neuropsychological battery and the patient-centred measures employed are described in subsequent sections.

The study was approved by the investigational review board of Galicia (CEIm-G, Santiago de Compostela, Spain) and signed informed consent was obtained from all patients prior to their enrolment.

2.2. Cognitive Functions

We assessed cognitive performance using the Brief Repeatable Battery of Neuropsychological tests (BRB-N) [15]. This battery includes several tests assessing cognitive domains: (1) verbal memory: Selective Reminding Test (SRT, with two subtests: consistent long-term retrieval as an indicator of consolidation, and delayed recall); (2) visual memory: 10/36 Spatial Recall Test (SPART, with two subtests: immediate retrieval and delayed recall); (3) attention and information processing speed (IPS): Symbol Digit Modalities Test (SDMT) and Paced Auditory Serial Addition Test (PASAT) with three second per digit version; and (4) semantic fluency and cognitive flexibility: Word List Generation (WLG).

Raw values were transformed into z-scores by adjusting for age and educational level according to the available Spanish normative data [16], and then grouped in terms of global cognition (zBRB-N) and for each cognitive domain. Failure in any test was considered when z-score was below -1.5 standard deviations (SDs) of the norm. CI in a given cognitive domain was defined as a failure in at least one test assessing that domain, and global CI was defined as an impairment in at least two cognitive tests evaluating the same or different cognitive domains. Patients without global CI were categorised as cognitively preserved (CP).

2.3. Patient-Centred Measures

Measures of HRQoL were evaluated using the physical and psychological components of the Multiple Sclerosis Impact Scale (MSIS-29v2) [17], a self-reported questionnaire ranging from 0 to 100 with higher scores indicating worse health, and by the Satisfaction with Life Scale (SWLS) [18], a five-item measure of self-rated assessment of subjective wellbeing scored from 5 (worst) to 35 (best). Symptom severity from the patient perspective was assessed by the SymptoMScreen questionnaire (SyMS), consisting of 12 items with higher scores indicating more severe symptom endorsement [19]. The Stigma Scale for Chronic Illness 8-item version (SSCI-8) [20] was used to evaluate internalised and experienced stigma across neurological conditions. It is composed of eight items and scores range from 0 to 40 with higher scores indicating higher levels of perceived stigma. Finally, the MOS Pain Effects Scale (PES) [21] is a 6-item self-report questionnaire assessing how pain and unpleasant sensations affect mood, capacity to walk or move, sleep, work, recreation, and pleasure of life. Total score ranges from 6 to 30, with higher results suggesting greater impact of pain.

2.4. Statistical Analysis

We described demographic, clinical, cognitive and patient-centred measures data by the median and interquartile range (IQR) for continuous variables and by absolute numbers and relative frequencies for categorical data. The normality assumption was checked by histograms and Shapiro–Wilk test. We explored differences in demographic, clinical and cognitive characteristics between AQP4-IgG-positive and -negative NMOSD patients using the Chi-squared and Wilcoxon–Mann–Whitney U-test or Student's t-test, when necessary, and demographic and clinical characteristics between CP and CI patients. Differences between patient-centred measures in previous groups were explored with analysis of variance.

We used linear regression to analyse the association between the z-score of global cognition (zBRB-N) and demographic (age and gender), clinical (disease duration, presence of AQP4-IgG antibodies, EDSS score, number of relapses before study inclusion, current treatment, BDI-FS and D-FIS scores), and patient-centred measures (MSIS-29v2, SWLS, SyMS, SSCI-8 and PES scores). We then fitted a multiple regression model including all the variables mentioned. We used the Akaike Information Criterion (AIC) to select the variables that best fit a model based on the whole cohort. For easier interpretation, all variables were standardised using the mean and SD.

In all analyses, we included age and gender as covariates to control for their potential influence on results. We used the false discovery rate (FDR) to correct for multiple comparisons, and we set the significance level to $p < 0.05$. All the statistical analyses were performed with R statistical software (version 3.6.0, www.R-project.org; accessed on 1 September 2021).

3. Results

3.1. Demographic, Clinical and Patient-Centred Measures of the Cohort

The demographic, clinical and patient-centred measures data of the 41 patients are summarised in Table 1. Patients were more frequently female (85%) and middle-aged (median of 44 years, IQR: 39–49), with a median disease duration of 8.1 years (IQR: 3.9–15.5) and a median EDSS score of 2.0 (range 0–7.5). Depressive symptoms were present in 18 (44%) patients: 12 (29%) had mild depression and 6 (15%) moderate depression. Four had concomitant disorders, one was also diagnosed with Sjogren's syndrome and three more with Lupus.

Table 1. Demographic, clinical and patient-centred measures data of the study population.

	NMOSD Cohort ($n = 41$)
Demographic and clinical data	
Age (years)	44 (39–49)
Female, n (%)	35 (85)
Disease duration (years)	8.1 (3.9–15.5)
AQP4-IgG positive, n (%)	27 (66)
EDSS score (range)	2.0 (0–7.5)
Number of relapses	2.5 (1–4)
Current treatment, n (%)	37 (90)
Beck Depression Inventory-Fast Screen (BDI-FS)	3 (0–6)
Fatigue Impact Scale for Daily Use (D-FIS)	6 (2–18)
Patient-centred measures	
Physical MSIS-29v2	35 (23–49)
Psychological MSIS-29v2	21 (14–29)
Satisfaction with Life Scale (SWLS)	21 (18–25)
SymptoMScreen questionnaire (SyMS)	16 (8–30)
Stigma Scale for Chronic Illness (SSCI-8)	9 (8–14)
MOS Pain Effects Scale (PES)	15 (9–20)

Qualitative data are presented by absolute numbers and proportions, and quantitative data by the median and IQR, unless otherwise specified. NMOSD: neuromyelitis optica spectrum disorder; AQP4-IgG: aquaporin-4 immunoglobulin G; EDSS: Expanded Disability Status Scale; MSIS-29v2: Multiple Sclerosis Impact Scale.

Twenty-seven patients (66%) were AQP4-IgG positive. The demographic, clinical and patient-centred measures data were not significantly different between AQP4-IgG-positive and -negative patients (see Supplementary Material Table S1).

3.2. Cognitive Characteristics in NMOSD Patients

Fourteen patients (34%) were classified as having global CI. Demographic and clinical characteristics were similar ($p > 0.05$) between patients regardless of their cognitive status. However, patients with global CI had lower satisfaction with life, more severe symptom endorsement, higher levels of perceived stigma, and greater impact of pain interfering with their lives than CP patients (Supplementary Material Table S2).

Figure 1A summarises the cognitive z-score distribution of each test from the BRB-N. Based on the definition of CI described above, the following frequencies of impairment in each cognitive domain were recorded: 10 patients (24%) in verbal memory, 14 patients (34%) in visual memory, 13 patients (32%) in attention-IPS and 3 patients (7%) in semantic fluency (Figure 1B).

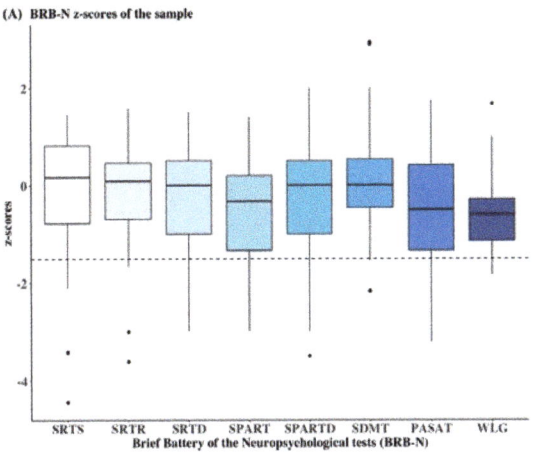

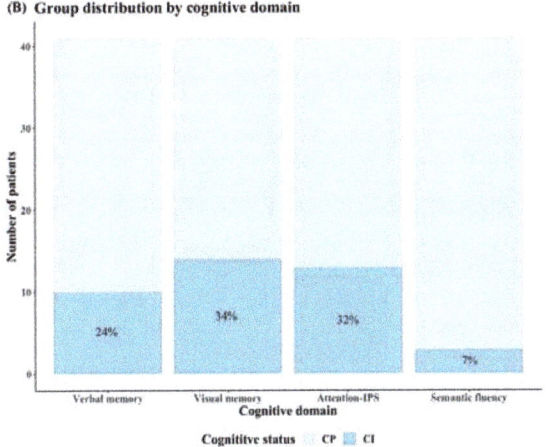

Figure 1. Cognitive performance in NMOSD patients. (**A**) Box plots represent the cognitive z-score distribution for each test from the BRB-N in the entire cohort; the *x*-axis depicts the name of each cognitive test and the *y*-axis the z-score for each test. The dotted black horizontal line represents −1.5 SDs of the norm. (**B**) The histograms show the proportions of patients with CP and CI in each cognitive domain. The *x*-axis shows the names of cognitive domains and the *y*-axis the number of patients for each domain. The total number of patients in each cognitive domain was 41. Both figures were fitted using R version 3.5.2 (R Foundation for Statistical Computing, Vienna, Austria). SRTS: Selective Reminding Test Long-Term Storage; SRTR: Selective Reminding Test Consistent Long-Term Retrieval; SRTD: Selective Reminding Test Total Delay; SPART: Spatial Recall Test; SPARTD: Spatial Recall Test Delay; SDMT: Symbol Digit Modalities Test; PASAT: Paced Auditory Serial Addition Task; WLG: Word List Generation.

When we analysed whether cognition was similar in AQP4-IgG-positive and -negative patients, we found no statistically significant differences in either the individual test z-scores of the BRB-N or the cognitive domains (see Table 2).

Table 2. Cognitive performance differences between AQP4-IgG-positive and -negative patients.

Cognitive z-Score	AQP4-IgG Positive (n = 27)	AQP4-IgG Negative (n = 13)	Corrected p-Value
Verbal memory			
z-score SRTS (storage)	0.17 (−0.49–0.86)	0.17 (−0.89–0.54)	0.952 [b]
z-score SRTR (retrieval)	0.23 (−0.60–0.50)	−0.25 (−1.08–0.46)	0.952 [b]
z-score SRTD (delayed)	0.0 (−1.25–0.50)	−0.50 (−1.0–1.0)	0.952 [b]
Verbal memory z-score	0.05 (−0.54–0.66)	−0.04 (−0.62–0.69)	0.977 [b]
Visual memory			
z-score SPART (storage)	−0.50 (−1.42–0.55)	−0.20 (−0.67–0.17)	0.952 [a]
z-score SPARTD (delayed)	0.0 (−1.5–0.5)	−0.50 (−1.0–0.0)	0.952 [a]
Visual memory z-score	−0.67 (−1.40–0.55)	−0.33 (−0.67–0.08)	0.952 [a]
Attention and information processing speed			
z-score SDMT	0.12 (−0.61–0.54)	0.0 (−0.29–1.29)	0.952 [a]
z-score PASAT 3	−0.50 (−1.29–0.65)	−0.44 (−1.33–0.33)	0.952 [a]
Attention-IPS z-score	−0.28 (−1.06–0.50)	−0.15 (−0.89–0.70)	0.952 [a]
Semantic fluency			
z-score WLG	−0.60 (−0.86–−0.18)	−0.6 (−1.17–−0.29)	0.952 [b]
Semantic fluency z-score	−0.60 (−0.86–−0.18)	−0.6 (−1.17–−0.29)	0.952 [b]
Global cognition (zBRB-N)			
BRB-N z-score	−0.32 (−0.93–0.21)	−0.17 (−0.97–0.15)	0.977 [a]

The data represent the median and IQR. AQP4-IgG: aquaporin-4 immunoglobulin G; SRTS: Selective Reminding Test Long-Term Storage; SRTR: Selective Reminding Test Consistent Long-Term Retrieval; SRTD: Selective Reminding Test Total Delay; SPART: Spatial Recall Test; SPARTD: Spatial Recall Test Delay; SDMT: Symbol Digit Modalities Test; PASAT: Paced Auditory Serial Addition Task; IPS: information processing speed; WLG: Word List Generation; BRB-N: Brief Repeatable Battery of Neuropsychological tests. The p-values were corrected by FDR adjustment. One patient was excluded due to unknown serostatus. [a] Student's t-test; [b] Kruskal–Wallis test.

3.3. Association between Cognition, Demographic, Clinical and Patient-Centred Measures

The global BRB-N z-score was associated with fatigue (D-FIS score: $\beta = -0.322$, 95% confidence interval, CI: −0.53, 0.12: corrected $p = 0.013$), physical impact of the disease on quality of life (MSIS-29v2: $\beta = -0.31$, 95% CI: −0.53, −0.09: corrected $p = 0.028$), satisfaction with life (SWLS: $\beta = 0.302$, 95% CI: 0.09, 0.51: corrected $p = 0.024$), self-perception of symptoms (SyMS: $\beta = -0.327$, 95% CI: −0.55, −0.11: corrected $p = 0.019$) and perception of stigma (SSCI-8: $\beta = -0.322$, 95% CI: −0.53, −0.12: corrected $p = 0.012$). Depression score was not related to cognitive performance (BDI-FS: $\beta = -0.188$, 95% CI: −0.41, 0.04: corrected $p = 0.306$).

Based on the AIC, the final multiple linear regression model included gender as well as depression (BDI-FS) and fatigue (D-FIS) scores, satisfaction with life and perception of the stigma (SWLS and SSCI-8). In our sample, 40% of the variability of the z-score of BRB-N was explained by this model (adjusted $R^2 = 0.396$, $p < 0.001$). A change of 1 point in the BDI-FS questionnaire, sensitive to depression, was associated with change of 0.6 points in global cognitive scores. Fatigue (D-FIS score), satisfaction of life questionnaire (SWLS) and perception of stigma for neurological diseases (SSCI-8) were also related to cognition (Table 3).

Table 3. Associations between the z-score of the global cognitive score (zBRB-N) and demographic, clinical and patient-centred measures.

Parameters	β (95% CI)	Corrected p-Value
Gender	−0.418 (−0.92–0.09)	0.102
Beck Depression Inventory-Fast Screen (BDI-FS)	0.654 (0.26–1.05)	0.002
Fatigue Impact Scale for Daily Use (D-FIS)	−0.388 (−0.72−−0.05)	0.024
Satisfaction with Life Scale (SWLS)	0.343 (0.08–0.60)	0.011
Stigma Scale for Chronic Illness (SSCI-8)	−0.361 (−0.65−−0.07)	0.016

Beta coefficients and 95% confidence intervals (CI) and p-values corrected by FDR adjustment.

4. Discussion

This study of a well-characterised cohort of patients with NMOSD diagnosed by the 2015 criteria shows that up to 34% of the patients suffer CI. Visual memory was the main cognitive domain affected, followed by attention-IPS and verbal memory. AQP4-IgG-positive and -negative NMOSD patients did not differ in their cognitive performance, despite having similar demographic and clinical characteristics. The study also identifies depression, fatigue, satisfaction with life and perception of stigma as the main factors related to global cognitive performance.

Although some attempts have been made to describe the cognitive profile in NMOSD patients, both the reported CI prevalence and the affected cognitive domains varied widely. Our results are in agreement with other studies reporting that around 34% of the patients can be classified as having CI [22,23]. However, the proportion of patients suffering impairment in our study differs from others with smaller cohorts [24–26], which applied different criteria for CI [6] or used other neuropsychological tools for cognitive assessment [27]. The most affected domain in our cohort was visual memory, followed by attention-IPS and verbal memory. These findings are in line with two recent reviews where memory, attention, and IPS are the most affected cognitive functions [5,8]. Similarly, Zhang and et al. found that both memory and IPS were more severely impaired in the visual than in the verbal spectrum [28]. Conversely, our results show a relatively preserved performance for semantic verbal fluency, which is one of the most pronounced dysfunctions in other studies [6,24].

We did not find an influence of clinical worsening, as measured by the number of relapses, disease duration and EDSS score, on cognitive performance. Moreover, no association was found between a positive AQP4-IgG status and cognitive performance, supporting the results of other studies exploring differences in cognitive test scores and APQ4-IgG status [28–30]. APQ4-IgG appears to inhibit neuronal plasticity, impacting the proper functioning of the glutamatergic system and water homeostasis by increasing excitotoxicity in cerebral grey matter [25]. However, this would not explain the CI observed in NMOSD patients who are AQP4-IgG negative. It is also unknown what causes the humoral immune response that produces the AQP4-IgG antibodies. Some infectious agents, even silent infections (*Mycobacterium avium* subspecies), have been involved in NMOSD aetiology [31,32]. Molecular mimicry between microbes and host peptides has been proposed as a mechanism that would exacerbate autoimmunity and generate autoantibodies. Interestingly, one recent study has shown a different pattern of humoral-driven immune responses against viral agents (HERV-W retroviruses family) between patients with NMOSD compared to patients with MS or MOG-IgG [33]. If such infectious agents could influence cognitive performance and its implication in autoimmunity deserve further studies. Additionally, the use of techniques such as non-conventional neuroimaging can shed light on the underlying mechanisms of cognitive decline in patients with NMOSD. In this regard, the presence of brain lesions at sites of high AQP4 expression, atrophy of deep grey matter structures or impairment of white and grey matter integrity have been proposed to be related to cognitive deficits in NMOSD [22,34]. It should be noted that the pathophysiological substrate of CI in patients with NMOSD is still not completely understood and should be further explored.

Mood disorders and fatigue are other major symptoms described in patients with NMOSD. We found a moderate association between fatigue and lower cognitive performance, while depression was not related to cognition. However, when we included fatigue and depression in the same model (after applying the AIC), among other variables related to HRQoL and gender, we found a strong correlation between depression and cognitive performance, suggesting a relationship between patients' psychological wellbeing and their performance on cognitive tasks. The relationship between depression, fatigue and cognition is not straightforward [1,29], but the current results indicate that the combination of both factors exerts a more deleterious effect on cognitive function. Overall, these findings highlight the importance of considering depression and fatigue symptoms in patients with NMOSD in the clinical setting.

Importantly, we found differences in the patient-centred measures between patients with impaired cognition and those with preserved performance. Indeed, in our cohort, we observed that patients with global CI had lower life satisfaction, showed more severe symptom endorsement, and perceived more stigma and pain. Moreover, when we analysed the association between patient-centred measures and cognitive performance in the whole cohort, we found that the global cognitive score was associated with the physical impact of the disease on quality of life, satisfaction with life, self-perception of symptoms and perception of stigma. These findings highlight the impact of cognitive and psychological impairment on the wellbeing of NMOSD patients.

This study has some limitations. First, the cross-sectional design did not allow us to assess the dynamics of the cognitive profile in NMOSD patients. Similarly, causal relationships between cognition and patient-centred measures could not be identified, and we were not able to add any pathological aspects related to brain damage in the linear regression analysis. In addition, although our cohort of patients with NMOSD is not very large, it is similar in size to other studies in this field and influenced by the low prevalence of the disease [29,35]. Further studies including more patients will be needed to explore the cognitive profile and the influence of clinical and pathological aspects on cognition. Nevertheless, our study also has several strengths. We described cognitive performance and its relationship with demographic and clinical characteristics and patient-centred measures in a sample of patients treated across 13 different hospitals throughout Spain, allowing results to be generalised to clinical practice.

To conclude, about 34% of patients with NMOSD included in our study had cognitive dysfunction, with visual learning and memory and attention-IPS being the most affected cognitive domains. Cognition was mainly associated with mood, fatigue, and the patient's positive attitude toward life and their perception of the disease. Cognitive and psychological assessments may be crucial to achieve a holistic approach in NMOSD patient care.

Supplementary Materials: The following supporting information can be downloaded at: https://www.mdpi.com/article/10.3390/jpm12050743/s1, Table S1: Demographic, clinical and patient-centred measures differences between AQP4-IgG-positive and -negative patients; Table S2: Demographic, clinical and patient-centred measures differences between CI and CP patients.

Author Contributions: Conceptualization, E.L.-S., S.L., R.G.-B., J.M., M.S. and E.S.; Methodology, E.L.-S., S.L., R.G.-B., J.M., M.S. and E.S.; Formal Analysis, E.L.-S. and E.S.; Resources, R.G.-B. and J.M.; Data Curation, J.E.M.-L., S.L., Y.B., F.P.-M., L.F., C.C., M.L.M.-G., I.G.-S., S.B., L.R.-P., Á.P.S., V.M.-L., L.Q., L.C.-F. and M.S.; Writing—Original Draft Preparation, E.L.-S., S.L., R.G.-B., J.M., M.S. and E.S.; Writing—Review & Editing, E.L.-S., S.L., M.S. and E.S.; Supervision, S.L., R.G.-B., J.M., M.S. and E.S.; Funding Acquisition, R.G.-B. and J.M. All authors have read and agreed to the published version of the manuscript.

Funding: This research was funded by the Medical Department of Roche Farma Spain (ML41397). The funders had no role in study design, data collection and analysis, decision to publish, or preparation of the manuscript.

Institutional Review Board Statement: The study was conducted in accordance with the Declaration of Helsinki, and approved by the investigational review board of Galicia (CEIm-G, Santiago de Compostela, Spain) (protocol code ML41397 on 27 September 2019).

Informed Consent Statement: Informed consent was obtained from all subjects involved in the study.

Data Availability Statement: Qualified researchers may request access to individual patient-level data through the corresponding author. The datasets generated during the analysis of the study are available from the corresponding author on reasonable request.

Acknowledgments: The authors would like to acknowledge all patients and their families for making the PERSPECTIVES-NMO study possible.

Conflicts of Interest: The authors declare the following potential conflict of interest with respect to their research, authorship and/or the publication of this article: E.L.-S. received travel reimbursement from Sanofi and ECTRIMS and reports personal fees from Roche, during the conduct of the study. J.E.M.-L. has received grants and consulting or speaking fees from Almirall, Biogen, Bristol-Myers-Squibb, Genzyme, Merck, Novartis, Roche and Teva. S.L. received compensation for consulting services and speaker honoraria from Biogen Idec, Novartis, TEVA, Genzyme, Sanofi and Merck. Y.B. received speaking honoraria from Biogen, Novartis, and Genzyme. R.G.-B. and J.M. are employees of Roche Farma Spain. F.P.-M. received compensation for serving on scientific advisory boards or speaking honoraria from Almirall, Biogen Idec, Genzyme, Merck-Serono, Mylan, Novartis, Roche, Sanofi-Aventis and Teva, outside the submitted work. C.C. reports personal fees from Biogen, Sanofi, Merck, Novartis, Teva and Roche, outside the submitted work. I.G.-S. has received funding for research projects or in the form of conference fees, mentoring and assistance for conference attendance from Biogen-Idec, Roche, Merck, Novartis and Sanofi-Genzyme. S.B. has received conference fees, mentoring, and assistance for conference attendance from Bayer, Biogen-Idec, Bristol-Myers Squibb, Roche, Merck, Novartis, Almirall and Sanofi-Genzyme. L.R.-P. received honoraria compensation to participate in advisory boards, collaborations as a consultant and scientific communications and received research support, funding for travel and congress expenses from Roche, Biogen Idec, Novartis, TEVA, Merck, Genzyme, Sanofi, Bayer, Almirall and Celgene. A.P.S. has received personal compensation for consulting, serving on a scientific advisory board or speaking from Almirall, Biogen, Bayer Schering Pharma, Merck Serono, Novartis, Roche, Sanofi-Aventis and Teva. L.Q. reports research grants from Instituto de Salud Carlos III—Ministry of Economy and Innovation (Spain), CIBERER, GBS-CIDP Foundation International, Roche, UCB and Grifols. He provided expert testimony to CSL Behring, Novartis, Sanofi-Genzyme, Merck, Annexon, Johnson and Johnson, Alexion, UCB, Takeda and Roche. He serves on the Clinical Trial Steering Committee for Sanofi Genzyme and is Principal Investigator for UCB's CIDP01 trial. L.C.-F. has received funding for research projects or in the form of conference fees, mentoring and assistance for conference attendance from Bayer, Biogen-Idec, Bristol-Myers Squibb, Biopas, Roche, Merck, Novartis, Almirall, Celgene, Ipsen and Sanofi-Genzyme. M.S. reports speaking honoraria from Roche and UCB Pharma, and travel reimbursement from Sanofi and Zambon. E.S. received travel reimbursement from Sanofi and ECTRIMS and reports personal fees from Roche, during the conduct of the study. The authors report no other conflicts of interest in this work.

References

1. Oertel, F.C.; Schließeit, J.; Brandt, A.U.; Paul, F. Cognitive Impairment in Neuromyelitis Optica Spectrum Disorders: A Review of Clinical and Neuroradiological Features. *Front. Neurol.* **2019**, *10*, 608. [CrossRef] [PubMed]
2. Weinshenker, B.G.; Wingerchuk, D.M. Neuromyelitis Spectrum Disorders. *Mayo Clin. Proc.* **2017**, *92*, 663–679. [CrossRef] [PubMed]
3. Lennon, V.A.; Wingerchuk, D.M.; Kryzer, T.J.; Pittock, S.J.; Lucchinetti, C.F.; Fujihara, K.; Nakashima, I.; Weinshenker, B.G. A Serum Autoantibody Marker of Neuromyelitis Optica: Distinction from Multiple Sclerosis. *Lancet* **2004**, *364*, 2106–2112. [CrossRef]
4. Wingerchuk, D.M.; Banwell, B.; Bennett, J.L.; Cabre, P.; Carroll, W.; Chitnis, T.; de Seze, J.; Fujihara, K.; Greenberg, B.; Jacob, A.; et al. International Consensus Diagnostic Criteria for Neuromyelitis Optica Spectrum Disorders. *Neurology* **2015**, *85*, 177–189. [CrossRef]
5. Eizaguirre, M.B.; Alonso, R.; Vanotti, S.; Garcea, O. Cognitive Impairment in Neuromyelitis Optica Spectrum Disorders: What Do We Know? *Mult. Scler. Relat. Disord.* **2017**, *18*, 225–229. [CrossRef]
6. Blanc, F.; Zéphir, H.; Lebrun, C.; Labauge, P.; Castelnovo, G.; Fleury, M.; Sellal, F.; Tranchant, C.; Dujardin, K.; Vermersch, P.; et al. Cognitive Functions in Neuromyelitis Optica. *Arch. Neurol.* **2008**, *65*, 84–88. [CrossRef]

7. Moghadasi, A.N.; Mirmosayyeb, O.; Mohammadi, A.; Sahraian, M.A.; Ghajarzadeh, M. The Prevalence of Cognitive Impairment in Patients with Neuromyelitis Optica Spectrum Disorders (NMOSD): A Systematic Review and Meta-Analysis. *Mult. Scler. Relat. Disord.* **2021**, *49*, 102757. [CrossRef]
8. Czarnecka, D.; Oset, M.; Karlińska, I.; Stasiołek, M. Cognitive Impairment in NMOSD—More Questions than Answers. *Brain Behav.* **2020**, *10*, e01842. [CrossRef]
9. Beekman, J.; Keisler, A.; Pedraza, O.; Haramura, M.; Gianella-Borradori, A.; Katz, E.; Ratchford, J.N.; Barron, G.; Cook, L.J.; Behne, J.M.; et al. Neuromyelitis Optica Spectrum Disorder: Patient Experience and Quality of Life. *Neurol. Neuroimmunol. Neuroinflamm.* **2019**, *6*, e580. [CrossRef]
10. Huang, W.; ZhangBao, J.; Chang, X.; Wang, L.; Zhao, C.; Lu, J.; Wang, M.; Ding, X.; Xu, Y.; Zhou, L.; et al. Neuromyelitis Optica Spectrum Disorder in China: Quality of Life and Medical Care Experience. *Mult. Scler. Relat. Disord.* **2020**, *46*, 102542. [CrossRef]
11. Meca-Lallana, J.E.; Prefasi, D.; Pérez-Miralles, F.; Forero, L.; Sepúlveda, M.; Calles, C.; Martínez-Ginés, M.L.; González-Suárez, I.; Boyero, S.; Romero-Pinel, L.; et al. Perception of Stigma in Patients with Neuromyelitis Optica Spectrum Disorder. *Patient Prefer. Adherence* **2021**, *15*, 713–719. [CrossRef] [PubMed]
12. Kurtzke, J.F. Rating Neurologic Impairment in Multiple Sclerosis: An Expanded Disability Status Scale (EDSS). *Neurology* **1983**, *33*, 1444–1452. [CrossRef] [PubMed]
13. Benedict, R.H.B.; Fishman, I.; McClellan, M.M.; Bakshi, R.; Weinstock-Guttman, B. Validity of the Beck Depression Inventory-Fast Screen in Multiple Sclerosis. *Mult. Scler.* **2003**, *9*, 393–396. [CrossRef] [PubMed]
14. Fisk, J.D.; Doble, S.E. Construction and Validation of a Fatigue Impact Scale for Daily Administration (D-FIS). *Qual. Life Res.* **2002**, *11*, 263–272. [CrossRef] [PubMed]
15. Rao, S.M.; Leo, G.J.; Bernardin, L.; Unverzagt, F. Cognitive Dysfunction in Multiple Sclerosis. I. Frequency, Patterns, and Prediction. *Neurology* **1991**, *41*, 685–691. [CrossRef]
16. Sepulcre, J.; Vanotti, S.; Hernández, R.; Sandoval, G.; Cáceres, F.; Garcea, O.; Villoslada, P. Cognitive Impairment in Patients with Multiple Sclerosis Using the Brief Repeatable Battery-Neuropsychology Test. *Mult. Scler.* **2006**, *12*, 187–195. [CrossRef]
17. Hobart, J.; Lamping, D.; Fitzpatrick, R.; Riazi, A.; Thompson, A. The Multiple Sclerosis Impact Scale (MSIS-29): A New Patient-Based Outcome Measure. *Brain* **2001**, *124*, 962–973. [CrossRef]
18. Pavot, W.; Diener, E.; Colvin, C.R.; Sandvik, E. Further Validation of the Satisfaction with Life Scale: Evidence for the Cross-Method Convergence of Well-Being Measures. *J. Personal. Assess.* **1991**, *57*, 149–161. [CrossRef]
19. Green, R.; Kalina, J.; Ford, R.; Pandey, K.; Kister, I. SymptoMScreen: A Tool for Rapid Assessment of Symptom Severity in MS Across Multiple Domains. *Appl. Neuropsychol. Adult* **2017**, *24*, 183–189. [CrossRef]
20. Molina, Y.; Choi, S.W.; Cella, D.; Rao, D. The Stigma Scale for Chronic Illnesses 8-Item Version (SSCI-8): Development, Validation and Use across Neurological Conditions. *Int. J. Behav. Med.* **2013**, *20*, 450–460. [CrossRef]
21. Stewart, A.L.; Hays, R.D.; Ware, J.E. The MOS Short-Form General Health Survey. *Med. Care* **1988**, *26*, 724–735. [CrossRef] [PubMed]
22. Kim, S.-H.; Park, E.Y.; Park, B.; Hyun, J.-W.; Park, N.Y.; Joung, A.; Lee, S.H.; Kim, H.J. Multimodal Magnetic Resonance Imaging in Relation to Cognitive Impairment in Neuromyelitis Optica Spectrum Disorder. *Sci. Rep.* **2017**, *7*, 9180. [CrossRef] [PubMed]
23. Kim, S.-H.; Kwak, K.; Jeong, I.H.; Hyun, J.-W.; Jo, H.-J.; Joung, A.; Yu, E.-S.; Kim, J.-H.; Lee, S.H.; Yun, S.; et al. Cognitive Impairment Differs between Neuromyelitis Optica Spectrum Disorder and Multiple Sclerosis. *Mult. Scler.* **2016**, *22*, 1850–1858. [CrossRef]
24. Vanotti, S.; Cores, E.V.; Eizaguirre, B.; Melamud, L.; Rey, R.; Villa, A. Cognitive Performance of Neuromyelitis Optica Patients: Comparison with Multiple Sclerosis. *Arq. Neuropsiquiatr.* **2013**, *71*, 357–361. [CrossRef] [PubMed]
25. Saji, E.; Arakawa, M.; Yanagawa, K.; Toyoshima, Y.; Yokoseki, A.; Okamoto, K.; Otsuki, M.; Akazawa, K.; Kakita, A.; Takahashi, H.; et al. Cognitive Impairment and Cortical Degeneration in Neuromyelitis Optica. *Ann. Neurol.* **2013**, *73*, 65–76. [CrossRef]
26. Yabalak, A.; Altunrende, B.; Demir, G.A. Cognitive Impairment in Neuromyelitis Optica. *Noro Psikiyatr. Ars.* **2021**, *58*, 200–205. [CrossRef]
27. Salama, S.; Marouf, H.; Reda, M.I.; Mansour, A.R.; ELKholy, O.; Levy, M. Cognitive Functions in Egyptian Neuromyelitis Optica Spectrum Disorder. *Clin. Neurol. Neurosurg.* **2020**, *189*, 105621. [CrossRef]
28. Zhang, N.; Li, Y.J.; Fu, Y.; Shao, J.H.; Luo, L.L.; Yang, L.; Shi, F.D.; Liu, Y. Cognitive Impairment in Chinese Neuromyelitis Optica. *Mult. Scler.* **2015**, *21*, 1839–1846. [CrossRef]
29. Moore, P.; Methley, A.; Pollard, C.; Mutch, K.; Hamid, S.; Elsone, L.; Jacob, A. Cognitive and Psychiatric Comorbidities in Neuromyelitis Optica. *J. Neurol. Sci.* **2016**, *360*, 4–9. [CrossRef]
30. Liu, Y.; Fu, Y.; Schoonheim, M.M.; Zhang, N.; Fan, M.; Su, L.; Shen, Y.; Yan, Y.; Yang, L.; Wang, Q.; et al. Structural MRI Substrates of Cognitive Impairment in Neuromyelitis Optica. *Neurology* **2015**, *85*, 1491–1499. [CrossRef]
31. Bo, M.; Niegowska, M.; Arru, G.; Sechi, E.; Mariotto, S.; Mancinelli, C.; Farinazzo, A.; Alberti, D.; Gajofatto, A.; Ferrari, S.; et al. Mycobacterium Avium Subspecies Paratuberculosis and Myelin Basic Protein Specific Epitopes Are Highly Recognized by Sera from Patients with Neuromyelitis Optica Spectrum Disorder. *J. Neuroimmunol.* **2018**, *318*, 97–102. [CrossRef] [PubMed]
32. Slavin, Y.N.; Bo, M.; Caggiu, E.; Sechi, G.; Arru, G.; Bach, H.; Sechi, L.A. High Levels of Antibodies against PtpA and PknG Secreted by Mycobacterium Avium Ssp. Paratuberculosis Are Present in Neuromyelitis Optica Spectrum Disorder and Multiple Sclerosis Patients. *J. Neuroimmunol.* **2018**, *323*, 49–52. [CrossRef] [PubMed]

33. Arru, G.; Sechi, E.; Mariotto, S.; Zarbo, I.R.; Ferrari, S.; Gajofatto, A.; Monaco, S.; Deiana, G.A.; Bo, M.; Sechi, L.A.; et al. Antibody Response against HERV-W in Patients with MOG-IgG Associated Disorders, Multiple Sclerosis and NMOSD. *J. Neuroimmunol.* **2020**, *338*, 577110. [CrossRef] [PubMed]
34. Blanc, F.; Noblet, V.; Jung, B.; Rousseau, F.; Renard, F.; Bourre, B.; Longato, N.; Cremel, N.; Di Bitonto, L.; Kleitz, C.; et al. White Matter Atrophy and Cognitive Dysfunctions in Neuromyelitis Optica. *PLoS ONE* **2012**, *7*, e33878. [CrossRef] [PubMed]
35. Chanson, J.-B.; Zéphir, H.; Collongues, N.; Outteryck, O.; Blanc, F.; Fleury, M.; Vermersch, P.; de Seze, J. Evaluation of Health-Related Quality of Life, Fatigue and Depression in Neuromyelitis Optica. *Eur. J. Neurol.* **2011**, *18*, 836–841. [CrossRef]

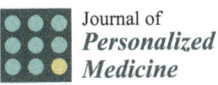

Journal of
Personalized
Medicine

Review

Towards Multimodal Machine Learning Prediction of Individual Cognitive Evolution in Multiple Sclerosis

Stijn Denissen [1,2,*], Oliver Y. Chén [3,4], Johan De Mey [1,5], Maarten De Vos [6,7], Jeroen Van Schependom [1,8], Diana Maria Sima [1,2,†] and Guy Nagels [1,2,9,†]

1. AIMS Laboratory, Center for Neurosciences, UZ Brussel, Vrije Universiteit Brussel, 1050 Brussels, Belgium; johan.de.mey@vub.be (J.D.M.); jeroen.van.schependom@vub.be (J.V.S.); diana.sima@icometrix.com (D.M.S.); guy.nagels@vub.be (G.N.)
2. icometrix, 3012 Leuven, Belgium
3. Faculty of Social Sciences and Law, University of Bristol, Bristol BS8 1QU, UK; olivery.chen@bristol.ac.uk
4. Department of Engineering, University of Oxford, Oxford OX1 3PJ, UK
5. Department of Radiology, UZ Brussel, Vrije Universiteit Brussel, 1090 Brussels, Belgium
6. Faculty of Engineering Science, KU Leuven, 3001 Leuven, Belgium; maarten.devos@esat.kuleuven.be
7. Faculty of Medicine, KU Leuven, 3001 Leuven, Belgium
8. Department of Electronics and Informatics (ETRO), Vrije Universiteit Brussel, 1050 Brussels, Belgium
9. St Edmund Hall, Queen's Ln, Oxford OX1 4AR, UK
* Correspondence: stijn.denissen@vub.be
† These authors should be considered joint senior authors.

Abstract: Multiple sclerosis (MS) manifests heterogeneously among persons suffering from it, making its disease course highly challenging to predict. At present, prognosis mostly relies on biomarkers that are unable to predict disease course on an individual level. Machine learning is a promising technique, both in terms of its ability to combine multimodal data and through the capability of making personalized predictions. However, most investigations on machine learning for prognosis in MS were geared towards predicting physical deterioration, while cognitive deterioration, although prevalent and burdensome, remained largely overlooked. This review aims to boost the field of machine learning for cognitive prognosis in MS by means of an introduction to machine learning and its pitfalls, an overview of important elements for study design, and an overview of the current literature on cognitive prognosis in MS using machine learning. Furthermore, the review discusses new trends in the field of machine learning that might be adopted for future studies in the field.

Keywords: multiple sclerosis; prognosis; cognition; machine learning; artificial intelligence

Citation: Denissen, S.; Chén, O.Y.; De Mey, J.; De Vos, M.; Van Schependom, J.; Sima, D.M.; Nagels, G. Towards Multimodal Machine Learning Prediction of Individual Cognitive Evolution in Multiple Sclerosis. *J. Pers. Med.* **2021**, *11*, 1349. https://doi.org/10.3390/jpm11121349

Academic Editor: Cristina M. Ramo-Tello

Received: 10 November 2021
Accepted: 9 December 2021
Published: 11 December 2021

Publisher's Note: MDPI stays neutral with regard to jurisdictional claims in published maps and institutional affiliations.

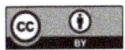

Copyright: © 2021 by the authors. Licensee MDPI, Basel, Switzerland. This article is an open access article distributed under the terms and conditions of the Creative Commons Attribution (CC BY) license (https://creativecommons.org/licenses/by/4.0/).

1. Introduction

As one of the most puzzling neurodegenerative disorders, multiple sclerosis (MS) is characterized by a complex biological etiology [1] and a highly heterogeneous disability progression. This gives rise to an important unmet need that has been given considerable attention in MS research in recent decades, which is the prediction of its future course [2–5]. In light of an ongoing paradigm shift in medicine, moving from a disease-centered to a patient-centered approach [6], the ability to foresee disability build-up in a specific patient would be a true game changer in modern medicine; neurologists could intervene at an early stage, whereas patients and their caregivers could anticipate future challenges in daily life.

Currently however, to predict the natural course of MS on an individual level remains challenging. Foremost, the problem is intrinsically difficult since the disease manifests differently among patients. From a biological point of view, tissue damage in the central nervous system (CNS), caused by auto-immune processes, is not restricted to a single location or to a particular timepoint during the disease course [7]. Typical observations are the presence of lesions, resulting from processes such as demyelination and inflammation, in conjunction with the loss of CNS tissue [7]. However, MS patients typically present a wide range of clinical symptoms as well, ranging from motor and sensory impairments to fatigue, cognitive problems, and mental health issues [8]. Since every person with MS presents a unique biological and clinical profile, health-related predictions should be individualized.

At present, the best tools to estimate individual disease progression are the so-called prognostic biomarkers. They are defined by Ziemssen et al., 2019, as: "A prognostic biomarker" that "helps to indicate how a disease may develop in an individual when a disorder is already diagnosed" [9]. Although these variables can be regarded as the cobblestones of the road towards an accurate prognostic model, it is important to note that this term is assigned regardless of any magnitude of prognostic accuracy. Moreover, they are typically established at group level, which might be a suboptimal fit in light of the aforementioned heterogeneity across subjects with MS.

In a recent systematic review by Brown et al., 2020, the authors identified several studies that used various statistical techniques to combine prognostic biomarkers [2]. Although the techniques used are widespread, some studies report on the use of machine learning (ML), allowing personalized predictions of the behavior of a clinically relevant variable over time. The literature on this topic was synthesized by Seccia et al., 2021, although the authors limited their search to models using clinical data [4]. As can be expected from a young field of research, a sprawl of underlying methodology is observed among papers that use ML to perform prognostic modelling in MS; heterogeneity in terms of input features, learning algorithms, labels to predict, and assessment metrics hamper comparability among models. The narrative nature of both aforementioned reviews underscores the fact that quantitative synthesis by means of, e.g., meta-analysis or meta-regression, is not yet possible. Furthermore, various models aim to predict disease progression in terms of changes in the Expanded Disability Status Scale (EDSS), while a recent review by Weinstock-Guttmann et al., 2021, questions the use of the EDSS for prognostic purposes due to a lack of accuracy and stability [3]. This review also highlights the importance to look at other domains, such as cognitive impairment [3]. Problems in various cognitive domains are prevalent in persons with MS, especially in memory and information processing speed [10]. Since cognitive functioning was shown to be related to socio-economic aspects such as employment status [11] and income [12], prognostication in this domain could allow patients and their caregivers to anticipate future problems at an early stage.

Although the use of machine learning for cognitive prognosis is still in its infancy, this paper aims to offer directions in this field by (1) introducing the concept of machine learning, (2) outlining the pitfalls of machine learning in medical sciences, (3) offering guidance for the design of studies that use ML for cognitive prognosis using lessons learned from ML-powered physical prognosis, (4) summarizing literature on ML-powered cognitive prognostication, and (5) highlighting trends in ML that could boost the field of MS prognosis. Since the main goal of this review is to provide directions for a young field of research rather than to synthesize the scarcely available literature, this review adopts a narrative, non-systematic design.

2. An Introduction to Machine Learning

Machine learning is defined in the Oxford University Press (OUP) as: "The use and development of computer systems that are able to learn and adapt without following explicit instructions, by using algorithms and statistical models to analyse and draw inferences from patterns in data" [13]. Although learning and adaptation can happen in multiple ways, typically categorized as "supervised", "unsupervised" and "reinforcement" learning, the most common machine learning technique adopted in the medical sciences is supervised machine learning. The notion of "supervision" here is the presence of the ground-truth label to be predicted, which can either be a continuous variable (regression) or a categorical variable (classification). In general, the goal is to learn the relationship, in terms of a function, between a given input and the output—the ground-truth label. The function that subsequently best predicts the ground-truth label on input data that was not used to learn the function is the model of choice.

The concept can be clarified by means of an analogy; a student studying for a future exam. In the first phase, the student will gather knowledge on the domain by using available resources such as books and lecture notes (training). The student subsequently verifies whether additional study is necessary by completing an exam from previous years to which the answers are available (validation). Together, this is called the training phase. As necessary, training and validation are repeated until the student is ready to take the final exam, which constitutes the testing phase.

Let us assume that we want to use supervised machine learning to predict a person's age given a brain magnetic resonance (MR) image. We start from a dataset with T1-weighted brain MR images (input) and the age at image acquisition (ground-truth label). Since age is a continuous variable, we are facing a regression problem. How we will learn the relationship between MRI and age depends on how we will use the MRI:

- Classical approach. The first approach is to analyze the brain MR images, yielding a set of features that describe the image such as volumetric quantifications of brain structures. This allows for the use of more classical supervised learning algorithms such as linear/logistic regression, support vector machines (SVM) and random forests (RF). Table 1 summarizes some frequently used supervised learning algorithms;
- Deep learning. The second option is to use the raw brain MR images as input and use a technique called deep learning, which recently gained popularity as a subtype of machine learning. The major difference compared to classical machine learning is that it mitigates the necessity to manually transform raw data in a meaningful feature representation, the so-called "feature engineering" step, relying on human domain-specific knowledge [14]. Deep learning will automatically create meaningful representations from raw data, thus achieving representation learning [14]. This will typically yield "latent features", which are hard to interpret by humans, but are deemed by the machine to be relevant. The advantage of deep learning lies in the more complex relationships that can be learned, while a major drawback is the need for large datasets, time and computational power.

Table 1. Supervised machine learning techniques exemplified for binary classification and univariate regression. For ease of interpretation, all examples use a low-dimensional feature space. However, the same principle holds when adding features towards higher-dimensional feature spaces.

Method	Description	Visualization
Logistic Regression	Logistic regression identifies the optimal sigmoid curve between the two labels to be predicted, yielding a probability of belonging to either of the two groups. In the illustration: the probability that a person will worsen or stabilize over time.	
Decision Tree	A decision tree is a sequence of decisions that are made on certain criteria. The last leaves of the tree indicate one of the class labels that are to be predicted.	

Table 1. Cont.

Method	Description	Visualization
Random Forest	This is an example of "ensemble learning", meaning that learning, and thus the resulting model, relies on multiple learning strategies, aiming to average the error out [15]. In this case, a random forest consists of multiple decision trees, mitigating the bias introduced by relying on one single decision tree. The ultimate prediction of a random forest classifier is the majority vote of the predictions of the individual decision trees in the random forest.	*Diagram: Decision Tree 1 → Worsening, Decision Tree 2 → Stabilizing, Decision Tree 3 → Worsening, Majority Vote → Worsening*
SVM	In case of two features, a support vector machine (SVM) tries to find a line or a curve that separates the two classes of interest. It does so by maximizing the distance between the line and the data-points on both sides of the line, thus maximally separating both classes.	*Scatter plot: Feature 1 vs Feature 2, with Worsening and Stabilizing classes separated by a line*
ANN	An artificial neural network (ANN) was inspired by the neural network of the brain and consists of nodes (weights) and edges that connect the nodes. Input data in either raw form or a feature representation enters the ANN on the left (input layer) and gets modified by the ANN in the hidden layers using the nodes' weights learned during the training phase, so that the input is optimally reshaped, or "mapped", to the endpoint that needs to be predicted on the right (output layer).	*Neural network diagram: Feature 1, Feature 2 → Input Layer → Hidden Layer → Output Layer (Worsening, Stabilizing)*
Linear Regression	Linear regression is a technique in which the weight of every input feature is learned, which is multiplied with their respective feature and summed together with the so-called "bias" (also a learned weight but not associated to a feature, i.e., a constant), yielding a prediction that minimizes the error with the ground-truth. In the 2D case, this is the line that minimizes the sum of the squared vertical distances of individual points to the regression line. The learned weights in this case are the slope (β_1) and intercept (β_0, bias) of the line.	*Scatter plot: Ground Truth vs Feature, with regression line $y = \beta_0 + \beta_1 x$*

3. Caveats for Machine Learning and Potential Solutions

Numerous pitfalls can be encountered when performing machine learning. The majority of them are generally applicable; they could arise in any machine learning query in any domain. Yet, we can encounter hazards that are specific for medical sciences. Both are discussed in this section, and solutions used in the field of prognostic modelling are also summarized.

3.1. General Pitfalls in Machine Learning

The most common pitfall in any machine learning query is overfitting. As already mentioned, a function is learned on training data and evaluated on validation and test data. Overfitting means that our learned function has become very specific to the training data, for example, because it also learned measurement errors in that dataset. Since measurement errors are different in another dataset, the function will be less accurate on that dataset. It is also possible, however, that we underestimate the complexity of the problem, which is the exact opposite case and understandably termed underfitting. For example, linear regression assumes a linear relationship between input features and the endpoint, which limits the model to only learn linear relationships, while the problem might be non-linear in reality. Figure 1 serves as a visual aid towards the understanding of under- and overfitting.

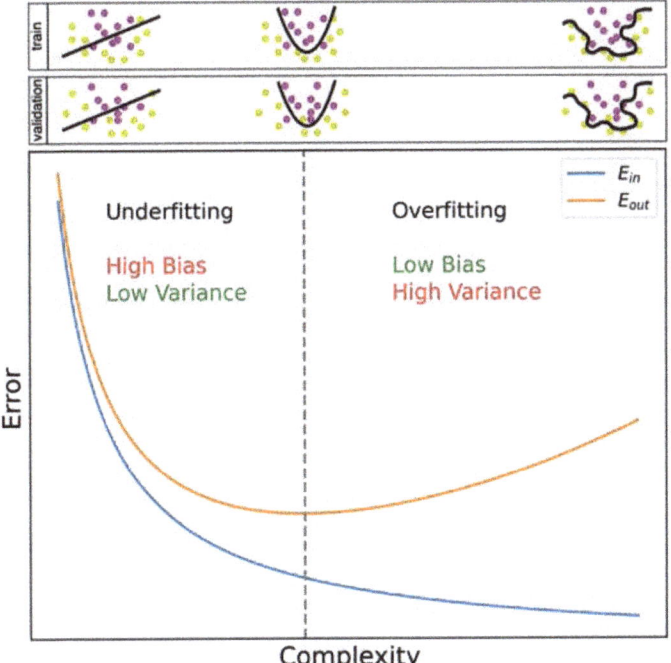

Figure 1. Bias–variance trade-off curve. Bias and variance vary according to model complexity [16]. The blue curve is E_{in}, the within-sample error representing the error on the training dataset. The more complex a function is allowed to be, the more specific the function becomes for the training dataset, i.e., overfitting. The latter is notable by the inception of an increase in E_{out} (orange curve, minimal value indicated with the vertical dotted line), the out-of-sample error, representing the error on the validation dataset. A simple function suffers high bias, i.e., it is highly likely to assume a wrong underlying function, since it only allows limited complexity between input and output to be learned (underfitting). By allowing more complexity, the bias decreases, but the function becomes highly variable depending on the dataset used for training (overfitting). An illustration is provided above, where the learned function is the line or curve separating two classes. From visual inspection, the optimal situation would be a smooth curve between the two classes (example in the middle). In the example on the left, underfitting occurs since only a straight line is allowed; many misclassifications occur in both training and validation data. In the example on the right, we observe a curve that squirms around all datapoints to fit the training dataset (overfitting), which, for example, happens when we allow the model to learn a complex function capable of learning measurement errors in a dataset. Hence, the function becomes specific to the training dataset; no misclassifications occur in the training data, but the same curve separating the validation dataset yields many misclassifications.

Overfitting often results from an imbalance between the number of variables and observations in the dataset. As a rule of thumb in the field, the number of observations should be at least 10 times as high as the number of variables [17]. To get to that ratio, we can address an imbalance in two ways: upscaling the observations or downscaling the variables. We note that in the case of downscaling variables, one should always remain vigilant not to underfit; informative features might be rejected as well.

1. Addressing the observations. Upscaling the number of observations is one way of tackling overfitting, but researchers often possess a database with a fixed number of observations. Nonetheless, several techniques exist to increase the number of observations based on those already present, e.g., using data augmentation. Although numerous variants exist, an easy-to-grasp data augmentation method is the insertion of random noise into an observation [18], and can be interpreted as a similar, yet different subject record. A generative adversarial network (GAN) [19] serves the same purpose, which we will explain by means of a metaphor. Imagine a game-like situation in which a radiologist has to find out whether an image is a true MR image of the brain or was produced by a computer, i.e., a "villain", trying to fool the radiologist. Initially, the radiologist will easily identify which images were produced by the villain, since it had no clue how to generate a representative image. However, since the villain receives feedback on its effort, it will gradually start to understand how to create an image that will give the radiologist a hard time in telling whether it is a true image or a fake one. The radiologist on the other hand is forced to keep on improving classification skills, since it gradually becomes harder to distinguish them, in turn stimulating the villain to propose better images. Hence, the radiologist and the villain will infinitely stimulate each other to perform better. Ultimately, MR images are produced by the villain that could in fact have been the true ones, and which can subsequently be used to expand a dataset. Similar to deep learning, a GAN needs, besides time and computational power, large amounts and diversity of data to create qualitative new observations;

2. Addressing the features. The second option to restore an imbalance is the reduction of the number of features that the algorithm will be trained on. In feature selection, only the features that are deemed informative are selected. For an outline of several feature selection techniques in the context of medical sciences, we refer to Remeseiro et al., 2019 [20]. The original set of features can also be transformed to a new set of features. This can, for example, be done with principal component analysis (PCA), where we could say that the features are "reordered"; an equal number of features are obtained—the "principal components"—that explain variance in the data in a decreasing order. Feature selection can then occur on principal components instead of the original features. The additional benefit of PCA is that it is a solution to the problem of multi-collinearity, in which features are mutually correlated. As a result, two variables might contain similar information, while the resulting principal components from PCA are uncorrelated [21].

Besides addressing observations and features, we discuss one additional technique to mitigate overfitting, which is training interruption. In their efforts to predict the progression of disease, Bejarano et al., 2011 [22] and Yoo et al., 2016 [23] stopped the training phase early by monitoring the error in the validation set. As can be seen in Figure 1, the error in the training set keeps reducing over time, since this is the goal of training. Initially, the same is observed for the validation data set, but upon obtaining a minimal value, the error will gradually increase, indicating the inception of overfitting. When stopping training at this point, overfitting might be mitigated.

Class imbalance is a specific pitfall for classification problems and is present when a certain class is overrepresented in the data, i.e., it contains more observations compared to the other class(es). For prognosis, subjects that do not worsen over time are often in the majority compared to worsening subjects [24,25]. Like overfitting, it can lead to the poor generalization of an algorithm [26]. Methods to correct class imbalance in a deep learning context are summarized in a systematic review by Buda et al., 2018 [26]. Two types of corrections are discussed, addressing either the data or the classifier itself. When addressing the data, we could restore the balance in two ways: by oversampling the minority class or by undersampling the majority class. On the other hand, we can make adjustments when training or testing the classifier. For example, one could decide to more severely penalize a misclassification towards a certain class compared to a misclassification towards another class, i.e., cost-sensitive learning [26]. These three methods were already explored in the light of prognostic modelling in MS to address the imbalance between stabilizing and worsening subjects [24,25].

3.2. Specific Pitfalls for Medical Data

Next to several general pitfalls, there are additional pitfalls when working with medical data:

1. Study data versus real-world data. Although the standardization of conditions and minimizing missing values are in general considered good practice, for example, when collecting data as part of a research study, it might limit the use of models in daily clinical routine that are known to be contaminated with, e.g., measurement errors, non-standardized test intervals, and missing values. When an algorithm encounters such inconsistencies during training, it could be expected to perform better on out-of-sample data. Although well-curated study data still dominate the field of prognostic modelling, efforts are underway to expand the use of real-world data [27,28];
2. Single-center versus multi-center data. This argument is similar to the former; data from different clinical centers might be different due to discrepancies in testing equipment (e.g., MRI scanner), testing protocols, and patient characteristics. Introducing this heterogeneity already during the training phase might increase generalizability;
3. Multiple visits of the same patient. Finally, when using multiple visits of a patient as separate observations in a dataset, one should always remain vigilant that the visits do not get intermingled between train, validation, and test datasets. Since visits are often highly comparable, the performance on an unseen test dataset could be biased, performing better than would be the case when adopting a truly independent test dataset. This could be categorized under the hazard called "leakage", in which information of the test dataset leaks in the training dataset. To prevent this from occurring, Seccia et al., 2020 applied a correctional method called "leave one group out" (LOGO) [27]. With this method, they withdrew all visits of one subject from the training set and used them as a test set, after which the procedure was repeated for all subjects. This hinders models to recognize patients within a dataset. Other methods were, for example, discussed in Tacchella et al., 2018 [29] and Yperman et al., 2020 [28].

4. Designing an ML Study for Cognitive Prognosis

Supervised machine learning is popular for its ability to provide personalized predictions on health parameters that clinicians are used to work with in routine practice. One of these use cases includes predictions on how a patient with a certain condition progresses over time (prognosis) [30]. In the following section, we will address relevant questions when designing a machine learning study for cognitive prognosis in MS, using a question and answer (Q&A) approach. Answers are mostly constructed using lessons learned from the literature on ML-powered physical prognosis in MS and the literature on cognitive prognostic biomarkers.

4.1. Which Outcome to Predict?

As mentioned before, the outcome (categorical versus continuous) will define the type of problem we are facing: classification versus regression. When looking at cognitive outcomes, the most commonly affected domains are information processing speed and memory [10]. According to Sumowski et al., 2018, information processing speed is best assessed with the Symbol Digit Modalities Test (SDMT), whereas for memory, the brief Visuospatial Memory Test—Revised (BVMT-R), California Verbal Learning Test—Second Edition (CVLT-II), and Selective Reminding Test (SRT) are the most sensitive tests [31]. However, composite scores also exist to provide a more holistic view on the cognitive status of persons with MS, which are summarized in Oreja-Guevara et al., 2019 [32]. In order to predict a change in these variables, a regression approach could include prediction of a future z-normalized test score [33], which is often the raw test score corrected for age, sex, and education level [33,34]. For classification, a popular categorization is defining "stable" and "declining" subjects [35], although wording can differ. In Filippi et al., 2013, for example, the authors defined cognitive worsening as an increase in impaired tests in a cognitive test battery over time, where impairment was defined as having a z-normalized test score below two [36]. Colato et al., 2021 defined worsening as a 10% decline of the SDMT score over time [37]. We furthermore note that practice effects can occur in cognitive tests over time [38]. To correct for this, a "reliable change index" was used in Eijlers et al., 2018 [35] and Cacciaguerra et al., 2019 [39]. Lastly, up until now, outcomes were all objective measures of cognition, while subjective, or self-reported measures also receive attention as outcomes for MS prognosis [40].

4.2. Which Features to Take into Account?

To be able to predict a future change in the variable of interest, the input of the machine learning model should receive careful consideration. Except when modelling on raw input data, learning should occur on features that are deemed informative towards the outcome to be predicted. To this end, we can use prognostic biomarkers, which were intensively studied in recent decades. However, although evidence on cognitive prognostic biomarkers exists, comprehensive reviews on the topic were mainly made for physical deterioration. We refer to reviews that summarize prognostic biomarkers for different modalities; demographics [41], clinical information [41], CNS imaging [42–45], molecular information [9], and neurophysiology [45]. Yet, there appears to be an overlap between physical and cognitive prognostic biomarkers. Although it is beyond the scope of this review to provide a summary of cognitive biomarkers, we refer to studies that identified cognitive prognostic biomarkers for different modalities such as demographics [35,46,47], clinical information [35,46,47], MRI [35,46,48], optical coherence tomography (OCT) [49], molecular information [50], and neurophysiology [51].

In analogy with the previous question on outcomes, subjective measures might also be informative for the prediction of disease course, such as patient-reported outcomes (PRO) [52]. Specifically for cognitive prognosis, features such as subjective cognitive impairment [47] and perceived ability to concentrate [53] were found to be informative.

4.3. On Which Time-Frame Should Predictions Be Made?

The literature usually makes a distinction between short-term and long-term prognosis. No clear cut-off between them has been reported, and this most probably depends on the clinical query that is addressed. Short-term prognosis is by far the most intensively studied [23,25,28], while Zhao et al., 2017 presented a longer-term predictive model of 5 years [24]. Yperman et al., 2020 stated that their rationale for a 2-year timeframe was based on maximizing the number of observations in the dataset [28]. Data availability is highly likely to hinder the field in performing longer-term predictions using machine learning, but studies investigating prognostic biomarkers for long-term disability already show promising results [36,46].

4.4. Which Machine Learning Algorithm to Use?

Given the heterogeneity in methodology throughout the literature, it is too preliminary to make firm statements regarding the superiority of one algorithm over another when considering performance. However, a second consideration is model complexity; linear models could underfit data, but are easy to interpret and familiar for clinicians. As illustrated by Sidey-Gibbons et al., 2019 [54], algorithms capable of handling increased complexity are in general harder to understand. This is, for example, the case for (deep) neural networks, which are often regarded as black box models [54].

4.5. How to Assess a Machine Learning Model?

Classifications will typically yield a so-called confusion matrix. In the case of a dichotomous endpoint, the confusion matrix is a 2 × 2 matrix with one axis indicating the true group labels and the other axis the predicted group labels. An example using the labels "worsening" versus "stabilizing" is illustrated in Figure 2, along with the metrics that can be calculated from this matrix. The different metrics allow us to study model performance from different perspectives. When looking at the confusion matrix of Figure 2, low sensitivity will leave worsening patients undetected, which causes neurologists to falsely assume that their patient is stabilizing. Withholding treatment—while this is in fact justified—will potentially endanger the patient's well-being. The opposite is true when we encounter low specificity; patients that do not worsen over time might receive treatment, while administration could potentially induce adverse events in their case.

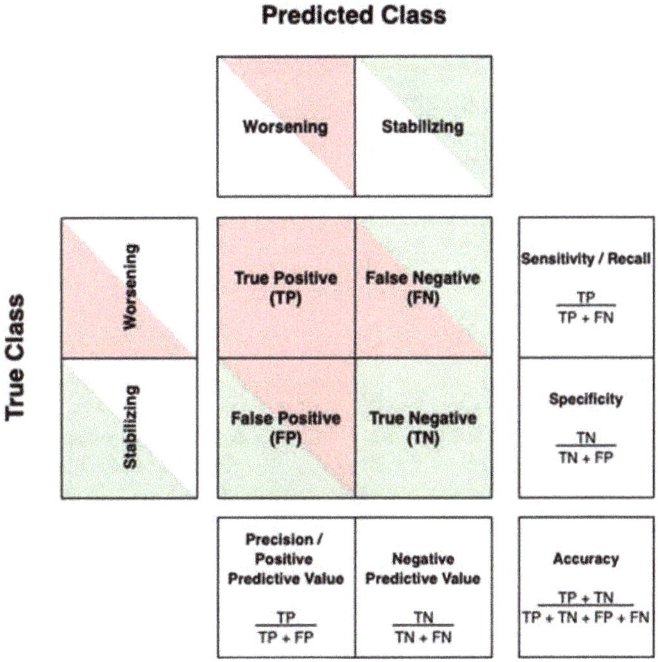

Figure 2. The confusion matrix and its derived metrics.

Regarding regression performance, the most intuitive metric is the mean absolute error (MAE); it represents how much on average the predicted value deviates from the true value, while making abstraction of whether this is an under- or overestimation. The main difference with related metrics such as the normalized root-mean-square error (NRMSE, RMSE [55], MSE) is that MAE retains the unit of the outcome variable. Other performance metrics include the correlation between the true and predicted outcome [56], the variance explained by the input features (R^2) [55], and the Akaike Information Criterion [55].

4.6. How Should Authors Report the Performance of Their Machine Learning Model?

Solid interpretation and comparability of models stands or falls with how papers describe their methodology and performance. As discussed in the previous subsection, different performance metrics give different insights in model performance. Although the importance of a given metric mostly depends on the domain context, it is essential to not only report scores such as accuracy, sensitivity, and specificity, but also present the raw confusion matrix in classification problems. For regression, a 2-column data frame with the predicted and true ground-truth label allows the calculation of measures such as the MAE, NRMSE, RMSE, MSE, and correlation coefficient. Providing such results in publications (e.g., in supplementary materials [27]) would be a leap forward in terms of reproducible research, while the anonymity of subjects remains assured.

The benefit is twofold. Firstly, the readership of machine learning papers can extract other metrics that they are interested in. Secondly, it would also allow future reviews on machine learning models to move beyond a narrative design. In systematic reviews for example, meta-analysis and meta-regression allows for the quantitative synthetization of data, which is possible since randomized controlled trials (RCTs) are strongly recommended to adhere to the CONSORT statement [57], guiding RCT authors towards correct, transparent, and complete reports. Although the CONSORT statement is not applicable to machine learning research, another statement in the "Enhancing the QUAlity and Transparency Of health Research" (EQUATOR, https://www.equator-network.org/, accessed on 8 December 2021) network is in fact applicable: the "Transparent Reporting of a multivariable prediction model for Individual Prognosis Or Diagnosis" (TRIPOD) statement [58].

4.7. When Is a Model Ready for Clinical Practice?

In order to introduce a predictive model in clinical practice, extensive technical validations and clinical performance evaluations are required, which should be complemented by ethical considerations and risk analysis. There needs to be maximal transparency towards the model's performance, so that regulators and clinicians can establish whether its error is acceptable in view of the potential risks to patients. However, when do we judge a machine learning model to be performant enough to be translated into a clinical decision support system (CDSS) [59]? In this regard, a first milestone is whether it performs better than random, but in a second phase, it should compare favorably against other potentially simpler models, such as decision rules based on single prognostic biomarkers. Among other factors, model complexity might influence the trust of clinicians in artificial intelligence (AI) [60]. Furthermore, it would be informative to know how the machine's prognostic accuracy relates to the accuracy of human prediction, in this case of the neurologist. Although the literature on the latter is scarce, we identified one paper on the accuracy of decoding cognitive impairment in MS, albeit cross-sectional [61]. The authors found the accuracy to be comparable to chance, and highlighted the need for improved cognitive screening [61]. In order to benchmark how a model would perform in similar conditions to actual clinical practice, study designs should directly compare the prognostic accuracy of medical professionals without and with the assistance of the considered CDSS. A typical scenario involves comparing whether the CDSS helps bridging the gap between medical professionals with different levels of experience. For instance, an ongoing trial investigates prognostic accuracy of junior and senior doctors in the domain of traumatic brain injury [62].

We note that although some models might be complex, several methods exist to enhance clinicians' trust. In Tousignant et al., 2019 [25], deep learning, which is currently one of the most complex machine learning algorithms, was used to predict worsening in EDSS from MR images. The authors used a two-step process to gain the clinician's trust, namely by quantifying the model's confidence in its own predictions, and verifying whether the model is correct when it is confident [25]. We note that a whole field of research, i.e., explainable AI (XAI), is dedicated to, among other things, augmenting user trust [63].

4.8. Which Data to Use?

To address this question, we refer back to the section on "Specific Pitfalls for Medical Data", where we discussed study versus real-world data, single- versus multi-center data, and dealing with multiple visits of the same subject.

5. State-of-the-Art ML-Powered Cognitive Prognostic Models

Literature in the field is scarce. This was confirmed by a PubMed search using the following search strategy: "(((multiple sclerosis[MeSH Terms]) OR (multiple sclerosis)) AND ((cognit*) OR (cognition[MeSH Terms]))) AND ((((machine learning[MeSH Terms]) OR (machine learning)) OR (artificial intelligence[MeSH Terms])) OR (artificial intelligence))", which was run on 3 December 2021, and yielded 39 records. Among those, we identified two studies that used machine learning for cognitive prognosis; Kiiski et al., 2018 [56] and Lopez-Soley et al., 2021 [64]. Kiiski et al., 2018 used supervised machine learning on different combinations of multimodal data, including demographic, clinical, and electroencephalography (EEG) data to predict short-term: (1) overall cognitive performance and (2) performance on information processing speed on a combined sample of persons with MS and healthy controls [56]. Lopez-Soley et al., 2021 also used multimodal data, including demographic, clinical, and MRI data, to predict short-term future cognitive impairment. This section is dedicated to the lessons that can be learned from their efforts.

Kiiski et al., 2018

First of all, the use of multimodal data is a good choice in light of the complex nature of MS and the identification of prognostic biomarkers in multiple domains. Moreover, the previous literature in the field of epilepsy established the superiority of multimodal data compared to using a single modality for machine learning predictions [65]. Secondly, the authors chose to z-normalize results for each neuropsychological test based on the mean and standard deviation (SD) of their sample, and use composite z-scores (average z-score of multiple tests) as the ground-truth label. A composite score was created for general cognitive functioning and one for information processing speed. Although transformation of raw test results allows comparison between, and aggregation of, different tests, the downside is in terms of clinical interpretation; clinicians have a reference frame for the original test results, whereas they do not for z-scores. Thirdly, the authors extracted over 1000 spatiotemporal features, whereas only 78 observations were used. This can be considered a large imbalance with a risk for overfitting, especially when considering the aforementioned rule of thumb of at least 10 times as many observations as features. The risk for overfitting might however have been reduced for several reasons:

- Using the "Elastic Net" [66] as learning algorithm. This is in essence a linear regression approach, but it uses regularization, which is the addition of constraints to the learning process to increase a model's generalizability. Specifically, it uses a combination of L1 (Lasso) and L2 (Ridge) regularization, which both tend to shrink large feature weights, whereas Lasso additionally tends to remove unimportant features from the model [66]. The low complexity of linear regression combined with regularization might have increased generalizability;
- Using cross-validation (CV), which is a technique that allows the use of data for both training and validation purposes by training multiple models. If no CV were used, only one model would have been created on a part of the data, whereas validation would happen on the remaining data. Since this is a balance between few data for training (risk for a poorly trained model) and few data for validation (risk for a poor evaluation of the model), CV is a useful technique to minimize both risks.

Fourthly, we previously mentioned the importance of benchmarking to obtain a reference frame for the quality of the prediction. For this, the authors created a "null model" by shuffling the ground-truth values across subjects before starting the learning phase. According to the authors, this provides an intuition in the "level of optimism inherent in the model" [56]. Lastly, we highlighted that using a combined sample of persons with MS and healthy controls increases sample size, but it obfuscates a clear interpretation of its value for prognosis in MS. Their best-performing model for general cognitive functioning included all available data modalities and yielded a mean cross-validated correlation of 0.44.

Lopez-Soley et al., 2021

Opposed to the regression approach of Kiiski et al., 2018 [56], Lopez-Soley et al., 2021 used a classification approach to predict future global- and domain-specific cognitive impairment [64]. The risk of overfitting was reduced by using Lasso regularization during logistic regression, 10-fold cross-validation, and retaining as much data as possible by imputing missing values.

Since cognitively impaired subjects were underrepresented for global cognition and all cognitive domains, it can be considered good practice that the authors used the "balanced accuracy" ((sensitivity + specificity)/2) to assess model performance across cognitive domains. The difference with accuracy (cfr. Figure 2) can be clarified with an example. Say that in a dataset, 20 persons with MS experience cognitive decline, and 80 do not. If the model correctly classifies 70 of the 80 stabilizing subjects, but only 5 of the 20 worsening subjects, the model achieves an accuracy of (70 + 5)/100 = 75%. The balanced accuracy, however is ((5/20) + (70/80))/2 = 56.25%. Hence, the balanced accuracy might be adopted for datasets that are unbalanced. For perfectly balanced datasets, accuracy and balanced accuracy yield the same value. Based on this metric, the authors reported the best performances for verbal memory (79%) and for attention/information processing speed (73%).

We note that by reporting the true class distribution, the authors greatly contributed to the interpretation of their result, as any evaluation metric can now be assessed with respect to that reference frame.

Overall, both studies yielded valuable intuition in the future design of machine learning studies for cognitive prognosis in MS. Despite the fact that predictions were obtained on a sample of both persons with MS and healthy controls in Kiiski et al., 2018 [56], predictive performances of both studies might serve as benchmarks for evaluating future studies in the field.

6. ML Trends and Opportunities for Prognostic Modelling in MS

Although studies dealing with prognostic modelling of cognitive evolution in MS are scarce, we see several interesting avenues for ML-driven prognostication in MS. We will discuss alternative approaches for prognostication, the simulation of treatment response and solutions to scarcity of longitudinal data.

6.1. Alternative Approaches for Prognostication

Hybrid predictions. Tacchella et al., 2018 introduced the proof-of-concept "hybrid predictions" [29] in the field of MS prognosis. The authors hypothesized that the discrepancy in "reasoning" between human and machine could in fact complement each other. Their results showed that the aggregation of human (medical students) and machine predictions consistently outperformed any of the single instances in predicting the conversion from relapsing–remitting to secondary progressive MS [29]. Besides performance, the fact that human intelligence is still involved in predictions could reassure clinicians that models do not solely rely on artificial intelligence, since they also rely on expert knowledge that algorithms might not be able to learn.

Digital twin. The field of machine learning for MS prognostication is mutually geared towards augmenting personalized care with personalized predictions. Since the prediction relies on the profile of a subject in terms of multimodal data, a subject can also be represented in a digital way, i.e., a digital twin. The concept of a digital twin was discussed elaborately in a recent review by Voigt et al., 2021, highlighting its potential to predict future disease course and simulate treatment effect [67].

6.2. Simulation of Treatment Response

Up until now, studies on prognostication mostly focused on predicting the natural course of multiple sclerosis. In our view, this is a necessary step to subsequently be able to predict, in a personalized way, how this natural course changes by administering certain treatment such as disease-modifying therapy (DMT). Although such estimates might be even more challenging, Pruenza et al., 2019 aimed to predict individual responses to 14 different DMTs [68]. The authors assigned a score per DMT that represented the likelihood of no disability progression in case of administration of the DMT [68]. Beyond a research effort, the authors created a tool that allows users to predict treatment response in new patients [68].

6.3. Solutions to Scarcity of Longitudinal Data

Transfer learning. A potential solution to scarcity of longitudinal data is to mitigate the necessity of building a model from scratch by using a robustly trained model from another domain, mostly related to the domain of interest. To this end, neural networks are typically used. Since the network's weights are meaningful to solve a related task, they could be used as initialization for the task of interest, updating the weights using a smaller dataset. For example, Nanni et al., 2020 used pretrained networks (trained on the ImageNet database [69]) to classify pictures of everyday objects (number of pictures in the order of millions), for prognostic purposes in Alzheimer's disease (number of MR images in the order of hundreds) [70].

Federated learning. For various reasons, data sharing in medical sciences remains delicate [71], which might explain why efforts in ML-powered prognostication remain largely single-center, extracting data from a single central database (centralized approach). However, an increasing number of studies [72,73] prove that machine learning can also occur in a decentralized way, i.e., by federated learning, meaning that data remain at their original location, while still being used for machine learning in a remote location.

Continual learning. In continual learning, an AI is not trained once, but evolves over time by augmenting performance along with the ever-going supply of novel data. The implications of this technique in medical sciences are nicely discussed in Lee et al., 2020 [74].

7. Conclusions

Machine learning is a rising concept in light of clinical decision support systems and personalized medicine and could boost the quest to find a suitable predictive algorithm for prognosis in MS. Investigations should however also address cognitive deterioration, and authors should be maximally transparent in reporting their results to allow comparison in the field. In doing so, clinical decision support systems using machine learning to predict future cognitive deterioration in MS could become a reality in clinical practice, providing the best possible personalized care for persons with MS.

8. Key Messages

- Machine learning is capable of handling multimodal data and could predict disease course on an individual level;
- The literature on cognitive prognosis using machine learning in MS is scarce. Future studies on machine learning for prognosis in MS should not overlook cognitive deterioration;
- Recommendations for the design of studies on machine learning for cognitive prognosis are proposed;
- Researchers should aim to share as many results as possible to allow benchmarking, solid interpretation, and comparison in the field, for example, by sharing raw predictions;
- Several trends in machine learning could overcome current roadblocks in ML-powered prognostic modelling in MS, such as scarcity of longitudinal data.

Author Contributions: Conceptualization, S.D., J.V.S., D.M.S. and G.N.; methodology, S.D., J.V.S., D.M.S. and G.N.; formal analysis, S.D.; investigation, S.D.; resources, S.D.; writing—original draft preparation, S.D.; writing—review and editing, S.D., O.Y.C., J.D.M., M.D.V., J.V.S., D.M.S. and G.N.; visualization, S.D.; supervision, D.M.S. and G.N.; project administration, S.D.; funding acquisition,

S.D., J.V.S., D.M.S. and G.N. All authors have read and agreed to the published version of the manuscript.

Funding: Stijn Denissen is funded by a Baekeland grant appointed by Flanders Innovation and Entrepreneurship (HBC.2019.2579, www.vlaio.be, accessed on 8 December 2021); Guy Nagels received research grants from Biogen and Genzyme, and is a senior clinical research fellow of the FWO Flanders (1805620N, www.fwo.be, accessed on 8 December 2021); and Jeroen Van Schependom is a senior research fellow of VUB.

Institutional Review Board Statement: Not applicable.

Informed Consent Statement: Not applicable.

Data Availability Statement: Not applicable.

Conflicts of Interest: Stijn Denissen is preparing an industrial PhD in collaboration with icometrix. Diana M. Sima is employed by icometrix. Guy Nagels is medical director of neurology at, and minority shareholder of, icometrix. The other authors declare no conflict of interest.

References

1. Winquist, R.J.; Kwong, A.; Ramachandran, R.; Jain, J. The complex etiology of multiple sclerosis. *Biochem. Pharmacol.* **2007**, *74*, 1321–1329. [CrossRef]
2. Brown, F.S.; Glasmacher, S.A.; Kearns, P.K.A.; MacDougall, N.; Hunt, D.; Connick, P.; Chandran, S. Systematic review of prediction models in relapsing remitting multiple sclerosis. *PLoS ONE* **2020**, *15*, e0233575. [CrossRef] [PubMed]
3. Weinstock-Guttman, B.; Sormani, M.P.; Repovic, P. Predicting Long-term Disability in Multiple Sclerosis: A Narrative Review of Current Evidence and Future Directions. *Int. J. MS Care* **2021**. Available online: https://meridian.allenpress.com/ijmsc/article/doi/10.7224/1537-2073.2020-114/471428/Predicting-Long-term-Disability-in-Multiple (accessed on 8 December 2021). [CrossRef]
4. Seccia, R.; Romano, S.; Salvetti, M.; Crisanti, A.; Palagi, L.; Grassi, F. Machine Learning Use for Prognostic Purposes in Multiple Sclerosis. *Life* **2021**, *11*, 122. [CrossRef] [PubMed]
5. Moazami, F.; Lefevre-Utile, A.; Papaloukas, C.; Soumelis, V. Machine Learning Approaches in Study of Multiple Sclerosis Disease Through Magnetic Resonance Images. *Front. Immunol.* **2021**, *12*, 3205. [CrossRef]
6. Lejbkowicz, I.; Caspi, O.; Miller, A. Participatory medicine and patient empowerment towards personalized healthcare in multiple sclerosis. *Expert Rev. Neurother.* **2012**, *12*, 343–352. [CrossRef]
7. Reich, D.S.; Lucchinetti, C.F.; Calabresi, P.A. Multiple Sclerosis. *N. Engl. J. Med.* **2018**, *378*, 169–180. [CrossRef]
8. Kister, I.; Bacon, T.E.; Chamot, E.; Salter, A.R.; Cutter, G.R.; Kalina, J.T.; Herbert, J. Natural History of Multiple Sclerosis Symptoms. *Int. J. MS Care* **2013**, *15*, 146. [CrossRef]
9. Ziemssen, T.; Akgün, K.; Brück, W. Molecular biomarkers in multiple sclerosis. *J. Neuroinflamm.* **2019**, *16*, 272. [CrossRef] [PubMed]
10. Macías Islas, M.; Ciampi, E. Assessment and Impact of Cognitive Impairment in Multiple Sclerosis: An Overview. *Biomedicines* **2019**, *7*, 22. [CrossRef]
11. Clemens, L.; Langdon, D. How does cognition relate to employment in multiple sclerosis? A systematic review. *Mult. Scler. Relat. Disord.* **2018**, *26*, 183–191. [CrossRef]
12. Kavaliunas, A.; Karrenbauer, V.D.; Gyllensten, H.; Manouchehrinia, A.; Glaser, A.; Olsson, T.; Alexanderson, K.; Hillert, J. Cognitive function is a major determinant of income among multiple sclerosis patients in Sweden acting independently from physical disability. *Mult. Scler.* **2019**, *25*, 104–112. [CrossRef] [PubMed]
13. Definition of Machine Learning. Oxford University Press. Available online: https://www.lexico.com/definition/machine_learning (accessed on 20 October 2021).
14. Lecun, Y.; Bengio, Y.; Hinton, G. Deep learning. *Nature* **2015**, *521*, 436–444. [CrossRef] [PubMed]
15. Polikar, R. *Ensemble Machine Learning*; Zhang, C., Ma, Y., Eds.; Springer: Boston, MA, USA, 2012; ISBN 978-1-4419-9325-0.
16. Hastie, T.; Tibshirani, R.; Friedman, J. *The Elements of Statistical Learning*; Springer Series in Statistics; Springer: New York, NY, USA, 2009; ISBN 978-0-387-84857-0.
17. Alibakshi, A. Strategies to develop robust neural network models: Prediction of flash point as a case study. *Anal. Chim. Acta.* **2018**, *1026*, 69–76. [CrossRef] [PubMed]
18. DeVries, T.; Taylor, G.W. Dataset Augmentation in Feature Space. *arXiv* **2017**, arXiv:1702.05538.
19. Goodfellow, I.J.; Pouget-Abadie, J.; Mirza, M.; Xu, B.; Warde-Farley, D.; Ozair, S.; Courville, A.; Bengio, Y. Generative Adversarial Networks. *Commun. ACM* **2014**, *63*, 139–144. [CrossRef]
20. Remeseiro, B.; Bolon-Canedo, V. A review of feature selection methods in medical applications. *Comput. Biol. Med.* **2019**, *112*, 103375. [CrossRef]
21. Jolliffe, I.T.; Cadima, J. Principal component analysis: A review and recent developments. *Philos. Trans. R. Soc. A Math. Phys. Eng. Sci.* **2016**, *374*, 20150202. [CrossRef]

22. Bejarano, B.; Bianco, M.; Gonzalez-Moron, D.; Sepulcre, J.; Goñi, J.; Arcocha, J.; Soto, O.; Carro, U.D.; Comi, G.; Leocani, L.; et al. Computational classifiers for predicting the short-term course of Multiple sclerosis. *BMC Neurol.* **2011**, *11*, 67. [CrossRef]
23. Yoo, Y.; Tang, L.W.; Brosch, T.; Li, D.K.B.; Metz, L.; Traboulsee, A.; Tam, R. Deep Learning of Brain Lesion Patterns for Predicting Future Disease Activity in Patients with Early Symptoms of Multiple Sclerosis. In *Lecture Notes in Computer Science (Including Subseries Lecture Notes in Artificial Intelligence and Lecture Notes in Bioinformatics)*; Springer: Berlin/Heidelberg, Germany, 2016; Volume 10008 LNCS, pp. 86–94. ISBN 9783319469751.
24. Zhao, Y.; Healy, B.C.; Rotstein, D.; Guttmann, C.R.G.; Bakshi, R.; Weiner, H.L.; Brodley, C.E.; Chitnis, T. Exploration of machine learning techniques in predicting multiple sclerosis disease course. *PLoS ONE* **2017**, *12*, e0174866. [CrossRef]
25. Tousignant, A.; Lemaître, P.; Precup, D.; Arnold, D.L.; Arbel, T. Prediction of Disease Progression in Multiple Sclerosis Patients using Deep Learning Analysis of MRI Data. In Proceedings of the 2nd International Conference on Medical Imaging with Deep Learning, London, UK, 8–10 July 2019; Volume 102.
26. Buda, M.; Maki, A.; Mazurowski, M.A. A systematic study of the class imbalance problem in convolutional neural networks. *Neural Netw.* **2018**, *106*, 249–259. [CrossRef] [PubMed]
27. Seccia, R.; Gammelli, D.; Dominici, F.; Romano, S.; Landi, A.C.; Salvetti, M.; Tacchella, A.; Zaccaria, A.; Crisanti, A.; Grassi, F.; et al. Considering patient clinical history impacts performance of machine learning models in predicting course of multiple sclerosis. *PLoS ONE* **2020**, *15*, e0230219. [CrossRef]
28. Yperman, J.; Becker, T.; Valkenborg, D.; Popescu, V.; Hellings, N.; Van Wijmeersch, B.; Peeters, L.M. Machine learning analysis of motor evoked potential time series to predict disability progression in multiple sclerosis. *BMC Neurol.* **2020**, *20*, 105. [CrossRef]
29. Tacchella, A.; Romano, S.; Ferraldeschi, M.; Salvetti, M.; Zaccaria, A.; Crisanti, A.; Grassi, F. Collaboration between a human group and artificial intelligence can improve prediction of multiple sclerosis course: A proof-of-principle study. *F1000Research* **2018**, *6*, 2172. [CrossRef]
30. Kourou, K.; Exarchos, T.P.; Exarchos, K.P.; Karamouzis, M.V.; Fotiadis, D.I. Machine learning applications in cancer prognosis and prediction. *Comput. Struct. Biotechnol. J.* **2015**, *13*, 8–17. [CrossRef]
31. Sumowski, J.F.; Benedict, R.; Enzinger, C.; Filippi, M.; Geurts, J.J.; Hamalainen, P.; Hulst, H.; Inglese, M.; Leavitt, V.M.; Rocca, M.A.; et al. Cognition in multiple sclerosis: State of the field and priorities for the future. *Neurology* **2018**, *90*, 278–288. [CrossRef] [PubMed]
32. Oreja-Guevara, C.; Ayuso Blanco, T.; Brieva Ruiz, L.; Hernández Pérez, M.Á.; Meca-Lallana, V.; Ramió-Torrentà, L. Cognitive Dysfunctions and Assessments in Multiple Sclerosis. *Front. Neurol.* **2019**, *10*, 581. [CrossRef]
33. Ouellette, R.; Bergendal, Å.; Shams, S.; Martola, J.; Mainero, C.; Kristoffersen Wiberg, M.; Fredrikson, S.; Granberg, T. Lesion accumulation is predictive of long-term cognitive decline in multiple sclerosis. *Mult. Scler. Relat. Disord.* **2018**, *21*, 110–116. [CrossRef] [PubMed]
34. Costers, L.; Gielen, J.; Eelen, P.L.; Van Schependom, J.; Laton, J.; Van Remoortel, A.; Vanzeir, E.; Van Wijmeersch, B.; Seeldrayers, P.; Haelewyck, M.C.; et al. Does including the full CVLT-II and BVMT-R improve BICAMS? Evidence from a Belgian (Dutch) validation study. *Mult. Scler. Relat. Disord.* **2017**, *18*, 33–40. [CrossRef]
35. Eijlers, A.J.C.; van Geest, Q.; Dekker, I.; Steenwijk, M.D.; Meijer, K.A.; Hulst, H.E.; Barkhof, F.; Uitdehaag, B.M.J.; Schoonheim, M.M.; Geurts, J.J.G. Predicting cognitive decline in multiple sclerosis: A 5-year follow-up study. *Brain* **2018**, *141*, 2605–2618. [CrossRef]
36. Filippi, M.; Preziosa, P.; Copetti, M.; Riccitelli, G.; Horsfield, M.A.; Martinelli, V.; Comi, G.; Rocca, M.A. Gray matter damage predicts the accumulation of disability 13 years later in MS. *Neurology* **2013**, *81*, 1759–1767. [CrossRef]
37. Colato, E.; Stutters, J.; Tur, C.; Narayanan, S.; Arnold, D.L.; Gandini Wheeler-Kingshott, C.A.M.; Barkhof, F.; Ciccarelli, O.; Chard, D.T.; Eshaghi, A. Predicting disability progression and cognitive worsening in multiple sclerosis using patterns of grey matter volumes. *J. Neurol. Neurosurg. Psychiatry* **2021**, *92*, 995–1006. [CrossRef] [PubMed]
38. Portaccio, E.; Goretti, B.; Zipoli, V.; Iudice, A.; Pina, D.D.; Malentacchi, G.M.; Sabatini, S.; Annunziata, P.; Falcini, M.; Mazzoni, M.; et al. Reliability, practice effects, and change indices for Raos brief repeatable battery. *Mult. Scler.* **2010**, *16*, 611–617. [CrossRef] [PubMed]
39. Cacciaguerra, L.; Pagani, E.; Mesaros, S.; Dackovic, J.; Dujmovic-Basuroski, I.; Drulovic, J.; Valsasina, P.; Filippi, M.; Rocca, M.A. Dynamic volumetric changes of hippocampal subfields in clinically isolated syndrome patients: A 2-year MRI study. *Mult. Scler. J.* **2019**, *25*, 1232–1242. [CrossRef] [PubMed]
40. Beier, M.; Amtmann, D.; Ehde, D.M. Beyond depression: Predictors of self-reported cognitive function in adults living with MS. *Rehabil. Psychol.* **2015**, *60*, 254–262. [CrossRef] [PubMed]
41. Degenhardt, A.; Ramagopalan, S.V.; Scalfari, A.; Ebers, G.C. Clinical prognostic factors in multiple sclerosis: A natural history review. *Nat. Rev. Neurol.* **2009**, *5*, 672–682. [CrossRef] [PubMed]
42. Louapre, C.; Bodini, B.; Lubetzki, C.; Freeman, L.; Stankoff, B. Imaging markers of multiple sclerosis prognosis. *Curr. Opin. Neurol.* **2017**, *30*, 231–236. [CrossRef]
43. Kearney, H.; Miller, D.H.; Ciccarelli, O. Spinal cord MRI in multiple sclerosis—diagnostic, prognostic and clinical value. *Nat. Rev. Neurol.* **2015**, *11*, 327–338. [CrossRef]
44. Davda, N.; Tallantyre, E.; Robertson, N.P. Early MRI predictors of prognosis in multiple sclerosis. *J. Neurol.* **2019**, *266*, 3171–3173. [CrossRef] [PubMed]

45. Leocani, L.; Rocca, M.A.; Comi, G. MRI and neurophysiological measures to predict course, disability and treatment response in multiple sclerosis. *Curr. Opin. Neurol.* **2016**, *29*, 243–253. [CrossRef]
46. Dekker, I.; Eijlers, A.J.C.; Popescu, V.; Balk, L.J.; Vrenken, H.; Wattjes, M.P.; Uitdehaag, B.M.J.; Killestein, J.; Geurts, J.J.G.; Barkhof, F.; et al. Predicting clinical progression in multiple sclerosis after 6 and 12 years. *Eur. J. Neurol.* **2019**, *26*, 893–902. [CrossRef] [PubMed]
47. Fuchs, T.A.; Wojcik, C.; Wilding, G.E.; Pol, J.; Dwyer, M.G.; Weinstock-Guttman, B.; Zivadinov, R.; Benedict, R.H. Trait Conscientiousness predicts rate of longitudinal SDMT decline in multiple sclerosis. *Mult. Scler. J.* **2020**, *26*, 245–252. [CrossRef]
48. Hildesheim, F.E.; Benedict, R.H.B.; Zivadinov, R.; Dwyer, M.G.; Fuchs, T.; Jakimovski, D.; Weinstock-Guttman, B.; Bergsland, N. Nucleus basalis of Meynert damage and cognition in patients with multiple sclerosis. *J. Neurol.* **2021**, *268*, 4796–4808. [CrossRef]
49. Bsteh, G.; Hegen, H.; Teuchner, B.; Amprosi, M.; Berek, K.; Ladstätter, F.; Wurth, S.; Auer, M.; Di Pauli, F.; Deisenhammer, F.; et al. Peripapillary retinal nerve fibre layer as measured by optical coherence tomography is a prognostic biomarker not only for physical but also for cognitive disability progression in multiple sclerosis. *Mult. Scler. J.* **2019**, *25*, 196–203. [CrossRef] [PubMed]
50. Gold, S.M.; Raji, A.; Huitinga, I.; Wiedemann, K.; Schulz, K.-H.; Heesen, C. Hypothalamo–pituitary–adrenal axis activity predicts disease progression in multiple sclerosis. *J. Neuroimmunol.* **2005**, *165*, 186–191. [CrossRef]
51. Nauta, I.M.; Kulik, S.D.; Breedt, L.C.; Eijlers, A.J.; Strijbis, E.M.; Bertens, D.; Tewarie, P.; Hillebrand, A.; Stam, C.J.; Uitdehaag, B.M.; et al. Functional brain network organization measured with magnetoencephalography predicts cognitive decline in multiple sclerosis. *Mult. Scler. J.* **2021**, *27*, 1727–1737. [CrossRef]
52. Brichetto, G.; Bragadin, M.M.; Fiorini, S.; Battaglia, M.A.; Konrad, G.; Ponzio, M.; Pedullà, L.; Verri, A.; Barla, A.; Tacchino, A. The hidden information in patient-reported outcomes and clinician-assessed outcomes: Multiple sclerosis as a proof of concept of a machine learning approach. *Neurol. Sci.* **2020**, *41*, 459–462. [CrossRef]
53. De Groot, V.; Beckerman, H.; Uitdehaag, B.M.; Hintzen, R.Q.; Minneboo, A.; Heymans, M.W.; Lankhorst, G.J.; Polman, C.H.; Bouter, L.M. Physical and Cognitive Functioning After 3 Years Can Be Predicted Using Information From the Diagnostic Process in Recently Diagnosed Multiple Sclerosis. *Arch. Phys. Med. Rehabil.* **2009**, *90*, 1478–1488. [CrossRef] [PubMed]
54. Sidey-Gibbons, J.A.M.; Sidey-Gibbons, C.J. Machine learning in medicine: A practical introduction. *BMC Med. Res. Methodol.* **2019**, *19*, 64. [CrossRef]
55. Kuceyeski, A.; Monohan, E.; Morris, E.; Fujimoto, K.; Vargas, W.; Gauthier, S.A. Baseline biomarkers of connectome disruption and atrophy predict future processing speed in early multiple sclerosis. *NeuroImage Clin.* **2018**, *19*, 417–424. [CrossRef]
56. Kiiski, H.; Jollans, L.; Donnchadha, S.Ó.; Nolan, H.; Lonergan, R.; Kelly, S.; O'Brien, M.C.; Kinsella, K.; Bramham, J.; Burke, T.; et al. Machine Learning EEG to Predict Cognitive Functioning and Processing Speed Over a 2-Year Period in Multiple Sclerosis Patients and Controls. *Brain Topogr.* **2018**, *31*, 346–363. [CrossRef]
57. Schulz, K.F. CONSORT 2010 Statement: Updated Guidelines for Reporting Parallel Group Randomized Trials. *Ann. Intern. Med.* **2010**, *152*, 726. [CrossRef]
58. Moons, K.G.M.; Altman, D.G.; Reitsma, J.B.; Ioannidis, J.P.A.; Macaskill, P.; Steyerberg, E.W.; Vickers, A.J.; Ransohoff, D.F.; Collins, G.S. Transparent reporting of a multivariable prediction model for individual prognosis or diagnosis (TRIPOD): Explanation and elaboration. *Ann. Intern. Med.* **2015**, *162*, W1–W73. [CrossRef]
59. Sutton, R.T.; Pincock, D.; Baumgart, D.C.; Sadowski, D.C.; Fedorak, R.N.; Kroeker, K.I. An overview of clinical decision support systems: Benefits, risks, and strategies for success. *NPJ Digit. Med.* **2020**, *3*, 17. [CrossRef]
60. Asan, O.; Bayrak, A.E.; Choudhury, A. Artificial Intelligence and Human Trust in Healthcare: Focus on Clinicians. *J. Med. Internet Res.* **2020**, *22*, e15154. [CrossRef] [PubMed]
61. Romero, K.; Shammi, P.; Feinstein, A. Neurologists' accuracy in predicting cognitive impairment in multiple sclerosis. *Mult. Scler. Relat. Disord.* **2015**, *4*, 291–295. [CrossRef] [PubMed]
62. Comparison of the Accuracy of the Neurological Prognosis at 6 Months of Traumatic Brain Injury Between Junior and Senior Doctors—Full Text View—ClinicalTrials.gov. Available online: https://clinicaltrials.gov/ct2/show/NCT04810039 (accessed on 2 November 2021).
63. Gunning, D.; Stefik, M.; Choi, J.; Miller, T.; Stumpf, S.; Yang, G.-Z. XAI—Explainable artificial intelligence. *Sci. Robot.* **2019**, *4*, eaay7120. [CrossRef] [PubMed]
64. Lopez-Soley, E.; Martinez-Heras, E.; Andorra, M.; Solanes, A.; Radua, J.; Montejo, C.; Alba-Arbalat, S.; Sola-Valls, N.; Pulido-Valdeolivas, I.; Sepulveda, M.; et al. Dynamics and Predictors of Cognitive Impairment along the Disease Course in Multiple Sclerosis. *J. Pers. Med.* **2021**, *11*, 1107. [CrossRef]
65. Memarian, N.; Kim, S.; Dewar, S.; Engel, J., Jr.; Staba, R.J. Multimodal data and machine learning for surgery outcome prediction in complicated cases of mesial temporal lobe epilepsy. *Comput. Biol. Med.* **2015**, *64*, 67. [CrossRef] [PubMed]
66. Zou, H.; Hastie, T. Regularization and variable selection via the elastic net. *J. R. Stat. Soc. Ser. B (Stat. Methodol.)* **2005**, *67*, 301–320. [CrossRef]
67. Voigt, I.; Inojosa, H.; Dillenseger, A.; Haase, R.; Akgün, K.; Ziemssen, T. Digital Twins for Multiple Sclerosis. *Front. Immunol.* **2021**, *12*, 1556. [CrossRef]
68. Pruenza, C.; Solano, M.T.; Diaz, J.; Arroyo-Gonzalez, R.; Izquierdo, G. Model for Prediction of Progression in Multiple Sclerosis. *Int. J. Interact. Multimed. Artif. Intell.* **2019**, *5*, 48–53. [CrossRef]
69. Deng, J.; Dong, W.; Socher, R.; Li, L.-J.; Li, K.; Li, F.-F. ImageNet: A large-scale hierarchical image database. In Proceedings of the 2009 IEEE Conference on Computer Vision and Pattern Recognition, Miami, FL, USA, 20–25 June 2009; pp. 248–255. [CrossRef]

70. Nanni, L.; Interlenghi, M.; Brahnam, S.; Salvatore, C.; Papa, S.; Nemni, R.; Castiglioni, I.; Initiative, T.A.D.N. Comparison of Transfer Learning and Conventional Machine Learning Applied to Structural Brain MRI for the Early Diagnosis and Prognosis of Alzheimer's Disease. *Front. Neurol.* **2020**, *11*, 576194. [CrossRef] [PubMed]
71. Van Panhuis, W.G.; Paul, P.; Emerson, C.; Grefenstette, J.; Wilder, R.; Herbst, A.J.; Heymann, D.; Burke, D.S. A systematic review of barriers to data sharing in public health. *BMC Public Health* **2014**, *14*, 1144. [CrossRef]
72. Brisimi, T.S.; Chen, R.; Mela, T.; Olshevsky, A.; Paschalidis, I.C.; Shi, W. Federated learning of predictive models from federated Electronic Health Records. *Int. J. Med. Inform.* **2018**, *112*, 59–67. [CrossRef] [PubMed]
73. Aledhari, M.; Razzak, R.; Parizi, R.M.; Saeed, F. Federated Learning: A Survey on Enabling Technologies, Protocols, and Applications. *IEEE Access Pract. Innov. Open Solut.* **2020**, *8*, 140699–140725. [CrossRef] [PubMed]
74. Lee, C.S.; Lee, A.Y. Clinical applications of continual learning machine learning. *Lancet Digit. Health* **2020**, *2*, e279–e281. [CrossRef]

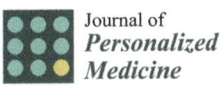

Article

Associations between Lifestyle Behaviors and Quality of Life Differ Based on Multiple Sclerosis Phenotype

Nupur Nag [1,*], Maggie Yu [1], George A. Jelinek [1], Steve Simpson-Yap [1,2], Sandra L. Neate [1] and Hollie K. Schmidt [3]

[1] Neuroepidemiology Unit, Centre of Epidemiology and Biostatistics, Melbourne School of Population and Global Health, The University of Melbourne, Parkville, VIC 3010, Australia; maggie.yu@unimelb.edu.au (M.Y.); g.jelinek@unimelb.edu.au (G.A.J.); steve.simpsonyap@unimelb.edu.au (S.S.-Y.); sandra.neate@unimelb.edu.au (S.L.N.)
[2] Menzies Institute for Medical Research, University of Tasmania, Hobart, TAS 7005, Australia
[3] Accelerated Cure Project for Multiple Sclerosis, Waltham, MA 02451, USA; hollie@acceleratedcure.org
* Correspondence: nnag@unimelb.edu.au

Abstract: Multiple sclerosis (MS), a neuroinflammatory disorder, occurs as non-progressive or progressive phenotypes; both forms present with diverse symptoms that may reduce quality of life (QoL). Adherence to healthy lifestyle behaviors has been associated with higher QoL in people with MS; whether these associations differ based on MS phenotype is unknown. Cross-sectional self-reported observational data from 1108 iConquerMS participants were analysed. Associations between lifestyle behaviors and QoL were assessed by linear regression, and phenotype differences via moderation analyses. Diet, wellness, and physical activity, but not vitamin D or omega-3 supplement use, were associated with QoL. Specifically, certain diet types were negatively associated with QoL in relapsing-remitting MS (RRMS), and positively associated in progressive MS (ProgMS). Participation in wellness activities had mixed associations with QoL in RRMS but was not associated in ProgMS. Physical activity was positively associated with QoL in RRMS and ProgMS. Phenotype differences were observed in diet and wellness with physical QoL, and physical activity with most QoL subdomains. Our findings show lifestyle behaviors are associated with QoL and appear to differ based on MS phenotype. Future studies assessing timing, duration, and adherence of adopting lifestyle behaviors may better inform their role in MS management.

Keywords: multiple sclerosis; lifestyle behavior; MS management; MS phenotype; quality of life

Citation: Nag, N.; Yu, M.; Jelinek, G.A.; Simpson-Yap, S.; Neate, S.L.; Schmidt, H.K. Associations between Lifestyle Behaviors and Quality of Life Differ Based on Multiple Sclerosis Phenotype. *J. Pers. Med.* **2021**, *11*, 1218. https://doi.org/10.3390/jpm11111218

Academic Editor: Cristina M. Ramo-Tello

Received: 4 October 2021
Accepted: 15 November 2021
Published: 17 November 2021

Publisher's Note: MDPI stays neutral with regard to jurisdictional claims in published maps and institutional affiliations.

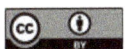

Copyright: © 2021 by the authors. Licensee MDPI, Basel, Switzerland. This article is an open access article distributed under the terms and conditions of the Creative Commons Attribution (CC BY) license (https://creativecommons.org/licenses/by/4.0/).

1. Introduction

Multiple sclerosis (MS), a chronic neuroinflammatory disorder, is commonly diagnosed in adults, predominantly women, aged 20 to 30 years [1]. On initial diagnosis, 85% of people with MS (pwMS) are diagnosed with relapsing-remitting MS (RRMS) presenting with acute attacks of new or increasing neurologic symptoms, and 10–15% with primary progressive MS (PPMS) defined by deterioration of symptoms from onset without obvious relapses or remission [2]. Within 15–20 years of diagnosis, approximately 50–75% of RRMS cases convert to secondary progressive MS (SPMS) defined by gradual worsening of neurologic function alongside a general cessation of relapses [3].

Both RRMS and progressive MS (ProgMS) may manifest an array of physiological, psychological, and motor symptoms; the number and severity of these symptoms and associated impairment play a critical role in quality of life (QoL). Symptoms of fatigue, pain, cognitive impairment, depression, and disability are key predictors of worse QoL up to 10 years later [4]. Improvement of symptoms through adoption of healthy lifestyle behaviors has potential to improve QoL.

Healthy lifestyle behaviors, including diet, vitamin D and omega 3 supplementation, and participation in wellness and physical activities have previously been found to be associated with higher QoL. PwMS who adhered to either high quality, MS-specific, or anti-inflammatory diets, have reported improved mental and physical QoL [5–7]. Vitamin D supplementation improved QoL in pwMS with initial levels lower than 30 ng/mL [8] and was associated with improved physical QoL in pwMS reporting an average daily intake of over 5000 IU [9]. Less is known about the effects of omega-3 supplement use, though in an international cohort of over 2500 pwMS, those self-reporting frequent fish consumption and taking omega-3 supplements had better QoL [10]. Research on wellness activity participation, ranging from Tai Chi and exercise therapy to mindfulness, relaxation, and imagery has mixed evidence of associations with QoL, though participation is generally reported to be beneficial for physical and mental QoL [11–14]. The benefits of physical activity for wellbeing are well established, with primarily aerobic forms benefiting social, physical, and mental QoL in pwMS [15].

Though the benefits of healthy lifestyle behaviors on QoL are evident, whether the effects are similar across MS phenotypes is unclear as most studies report on populations of mixed phenotype. As people with ProgMS are generally less responsive to therapies, have greater disability and more severe symptoms than those with RRMS [16–18], it is probable that the effects of lifestyle behaviors on QoL also differ. Therefore, we aim to differentiate associations of lifestyle behaviors with QoL between phenotypes, which may provide insight into personalised management strategies specific to disease course.

2. Materials and Methods

2.1. Study Design and Participants

Commencing from 2014, recruitment to the iConquerMS observational study has been ongoing and open to pwMS and the general population aged ≥21 years. The study is promoted by the sponsoring organization, Accelerated Cure Project for MS, and partner organizations and individuals via online, print and in person communication. Consenting participants are requested to voluntarily complete a series of self-reported online surveys capturing demographics, health and clinical outcomes, as well as lifestyle behaviors, at 6 month intervals. Response to questions at any timepoint is optional.

De-identified baseline data from participants who registered in the study from November 2014 to July 2020 (n = 3374) was extracted. Inclusion criteria were participants reporting a clinician-confirmed MS diagnosis, confidence in MS diagnosis, and having completed diet and wellness, physical activity, QoL and disability surveys. RRMS, SPMS or PPMS phenotypes were included, and SPMS/PPMS consolidated. Clinically isolated syndrome, radiologically isolated syndrome, and not sure/don't know MS phenotype, were excluded. Ethics approval ID #1956113.1.

2.2. Demographics and Clinical Outcomes

Age (from date of birth), sex (male, female), highest level of education (no formal education, elementary-middle school, high school, high school graduate, some college, associate degree, technical degree, bachelor's degree, master's degree, doctoral degree), partner status (never married, married, divorced, separated, widowed, cohabitation/domestic partner, prefer not to answer), employment status (employed outside home, employed at home, homemaker, student, worker's compensation, unemployed looking for work, disabled), country of birth (global country list), ethnicity (American Indian/Alaska Native, Middle Eastern, South Asian, other Asian, Black/African American, Native Hawaiian/Pacific Islander, White, don't know), and annual household income (<USD15,000 to >USD200,001 in increments of USD15,000) were queried and re-categorized.

MS duration was calculated by year of diagnosis and survey completion. Body mass index (BMI) was calculated by weight (kg)/height (m)^2 then categorized into underweight, normal, overweight, and obese according to World Health Organisation classifications [19]; underweight and normal were combined due to small sample size in the former group. Disability was measured via the Patient Determined Disease Steps (PDDS), and scores collapsed to low (0–2), moderate (3–5) and high (6–8) disability as per guidelines [20].

2.3. Lifestyle Behaviors

Variables within diet (*n* = 23), wellness (*n* = 25), vitamins (*n* = 15) and supplements (*n* = 29) categories were each queried via tick-box options of "used" and/or "used and helpful" in the past 6 months to improve health and wellbeing; those not selecting either were considered not using. Two response options were combined for analysis (Yes = used/used and helpful vs. No = none selected). Variables were recategorized for diet and wellness (Table 1) then analysed as a binary variable (Yes = use/used and helpful of $\geq$1 option within category). Of the vitamins and supplements, only vitamin D and omega-3 were analysed.

Table 1. Lifestyle Behavior Categories.

Lifestyle	Category	Inclusions
Diet	Anti-inflammatory	Anti-inflammatory, fasting/calorie restriction, gluten-free, Mediterranean
	Low-saturated fats	Jelinek, Swank, low-fat, ovo-lactovegetarian, vegetarian, vegan, lacto-vegetarian, Ornish, Pritikin, pescatarian
	Low-carbohydrate	Atkins, ketogenic, paleo, Wahls, low-carbohydrate
	Other	Organic, low sodium, low sugar, semi-vegetarian
Supplements	Vitamin D	Vitamin D
	Omega-3	Omega-3, DHA or EPA fatty acid, fish-oil, flaxseed/flaxseed oil
Wellness	Mind	Meditation, mindfulness, guided imagery, relaxation exercise, stress management
	Mind-body	Tai chi, yoga, qigong, exercise therapy
	Other	Acupuncture, Ayurveda, biofeedback, brain training, chelation therapy, chiropractic/osteopathic manipulation, cognitive behavioral therapy, craniosacral therapy, deep breathing exercises, energy healing, hypnosis, massage, naturopathy, progressive relaxation, reflexology, traditional healing
Physical activity	Sedentary	leisure activity score <14
	Moderate	leisure activity score 14–23
	Active	leisure activity score >23

Physical activity was assessed via the Godin-Shephard Leisure-Time Physical Activity Questionnaire (GLTPAQ), which queries frequency (0–7 days) of strenuous, moderate, and mild exercise for $\geq$ 15 min in the preceding seven days [21]. Total leisure activity score was calculated as per guidelines and categorized into sedentary (<14), moderately active (14–23), and active ($\geq$24).

2.4. Outcome Measure

QoL was queried via the NeuroQoL Adult Short Form, comprising 13 subdomains, classified under physical, mental, and social QoL [22]. Each of 13 subdomains comprise between five to nine questions scored on a Likert scale. Scores were summated and converted to T-scores (Mean = 50, SD = 10) as per guidelines. For mobility, fine motor, anxiety, depression, positive affect, cognitive function, social participation, and social satisfaction subdomains, T-scores were derived from an average U.S. general population; and for fatigue, sleep disturbance, emotional dyscontrol, and stigma subdomains, T-scores were derived from an average population with a diagnosed neurological disorder (MS, epilepsy, stroke, amyotrophic lateral sclerosis, or Parkinson's disease). Higher T-scores equate to higher measured concept. T-scores for the communication subdomain were unavailable, therefore raw total score for this subdomain was used for analysis and reporting.

2.5. Statistical Analysis

All analyses were conducted in Stata version 15.0 (StataCorp. 2017. Stata Statistical Software: Release 15. College Station, TX, USA: StataCorp LLC.). Associations between lifestyle behavior categories and QoL domain were assessed by multiple linear regression models, adjusted for age, sex, education, BMI, disability, and duration since MS diagnosis, estimating adjusted regression coefficients and 95% CI. An interaction term between

MS phenotype and each lifestyle behavior was added to the regression model to assess differences between RRMS and ProgMS.

3. Results

3.1. Participant Characteristics Based on Phenotype

Of 3374 participants enrolled into iConquerMS, $n = 1108$ (33%) met the inclusion criteria. In the included population, compared to participants with RRMS, people with ProgMS were older, and more likely to be male, not in paid employment, with moderate or severe disability, and longer MS duration (Table 2A). For lifestyle behaviors, compared to RRMS, people with ProgMS were less likely to have used an anti-inflammatory diet, and less likely to be at an active level of physical activity.

Table 2. (**A**). Characteristics of participants with RRMS and ProgMS. (**B**). Mean QoL T-scores of participants with RRMS and ProgMS.

(A)								
Demographics	RRMS $n = 750$	ProgMS $n = 358$	*p*	Lifestyle Behaviors	RRMS $n = 750$	ProgMS $n = 358$	*p*
	n (%)	n (%)			n (%)	n (%)	
Age, years (Mean, SD)	49.9 (11)	58.3 (9)	<0.001	Diet			
Sex				Anti-inflammatory			
Male	126 (17%)	113 (32%)	Ref.	Not used	464 (62%)	245 (68%)	Ref.
Female	621 (83%)	244 (68%)	<0.001	Used/helpful	286 (38%)	113 (32%)	<0.05
Country of birth				Low saturated fat			
US	634 (85%)	308 (86%)	Ref.	Not used	601 (80%)	300 (84%)	Ref.
Other	114 (15%)	50 (14%)	0.59	Used/helpful	149 (20%)	58 (16%)	0.16
Ethnicity				Low carbohydrate			
Caucasian	688 (92%)	337 (95%)	Ref.	Not used	576 (77%)	280 (78%)	Ref.
Other/mixed	56 (8%)	18 (5%)	0.15	Used/helpful	174 (23%)	78 (22%)	0.61
University degree				Other			
Yes	525 (70%)	245 (68%)	Ref.	Not used	500 (67%)	252 (70%)	Ref.
No	222 (30%)	113 (32%)	0.55	Used/helpful	250 (33%)	106 (30%)	0.23
Partnered				Supplements			
Yes	530 (71%)	274 (77%)	Ref.	Vitamin D			
No	214 (29%)	84 (24%)	0.06	No	108 (14%)	65 (18%)	Ref.
Paid employment				Yes	642 (86%)	293 (82%)	0.10
Yes	402 (54%)	94 (27%)	Ref.	Omega-3			
No	338 (46%)	260 (74%)	<0.001	Not used	461 (61%)	210 (59%)	Ref.
Household income (USD)				Used/helpful	289 (39%)	148 (41%)	0.36
≤$50,000	144 (35%)	67 (42%)	Ref.	**Wellness**			
$50,001–100,000	121 (29%)	49 (31%)	0.56	Mind			
≥$100,001	146 (35%)	44 (28%)	0.06	Not used	473 (63%)	231 (65%)	Ref.
BMI				Used/helpful	277 (37%)	127 (36%)	0.65
Under/healthy	331 (44%)	166 (47%)	Ref.	Mind-body			
Overweight	204 (27%)	103 (29%)	0.99	Not used	456 (61%)	224 (63%)	Ref.
Obese	212 (28%)	86 (24%)	0.19	Used/helpful	294 (39%)	134 (37%)	0.58
PDDS				Other			
Normal/mild	448 (60%)	36 (10%)	Ref.	Not used	249 (33%)	132 (37%)	Ref.

Table 2. Cont.

(A)

Demographics	RRMS n = 750	ProgMS n = 358	p	Lifestyle Behaviors	RRMS n = 750	ProgMS n = 358	p
	n (%)	n (%)			n (%)	n (%)	
Moderate	252 (34%)	186 (52%)	<0.001	Used/helpful Physical activity	501 (67%)	226 (63%)	0.24
Severe	50 (7%)	135 (38%)	<0.001				
MS duration (years)	11.5 (9.1)	16.1 (10.3)	<0.001	Sedentary	225 (30%)	154 (43%)	Ref.
				Moderate	150 (20%)	84 (24%)	0.25
				Active	375 (50%)	120 (34%)	<0.001

(B)

QoL Subdomains	RRMS n = 750	ProgMS n = 358	p
	Mean (SD) T-score	Mean (SD) T-score	
Physical			
Mobility	48.0 (9.0)	**38.30 (7.5)**	<0.001
Fine motor	46.4 (8.7)	41.0 (9.2)	<0.001
Fatigue	51.8 (9.5)	53.3 (8.5)	<0.05
Sleep disturbance	53.8 (9.0)	53.4 (7.8)	0.433
Mental			
Anxiety	51.8 (8.6)	50.6 (7.6)	<0.05
Depression	47.7 (8.3)	48.4 (7.9)	0.185
Positive affect	52.5 (8.2)	51.1 (8.1)	<0.01
Emotional dyscontrol	48.6 (9.8)	48.1 (9.2)	0.394
Stigma	49.0 (7.8)	52.7 (6.9)	<0.001
Cognitive function	45.8 (10.7)	46.6 (10.2)	0.259
Communication [a]	22.1 (3.4)	21.9 (3.5)	0.390
Social			
Participation	46.8 (7.9)	43.7 (6.4)	<0.001
Satisfaction	45.3 (7.0)	42.0 (5.5)	<0.001

BMI = body mass index; MS = multiple sclerosis; PDSS = Patient Determined Disease Steps; ProgMS = progressive MS; Ref. = reference; RRMS = relapsing-remitting MS; SD = standard deviation; USD = United States Dollar. p values indicate statistical differences between RRMS and ProgMS, where bolded values indicate significance ($p < 0.05$). [a] Total raw score. Bolded mean scores indicate differences > 5 points on the T-scale metric (0.5 SD) than the clinical or US general population.

For QoL, compared to the clinical for U.S. general population, pwMS reported similar T-score difference (<0.5 SD) in 9 of 13 QoL subdomains, excepting fine motor, mobility, and both social participation and satisfaction (Table 2B), in which people with ProgMS reported marginally lower T-scores. Compared to RRMS, people with ProgMS reported significantly worse QoL in 7 of 13 subdomains: lower mobility, fine motor, positive affect, and both social participation and satisfaction, and higher fatigue and stigma. Anxiety was higher in RRMS (Table 2B).

3.2. Associations between Lifestyle and Quality of Life Subdomains

Diet was associated with physical and mental, but not social, QoL (Table 3A). In people with RRMS, anti-inflammatory, low-carbohydrate and other diets were positively associated with stigma, and other diets additionally associated with lower fine motor and cognitive function. In ProgMS, anti-inflammatory diets were associated with higher mobility and positive affect; low-carbohydrate diet with higher positive affect; low-saturated fat diet with higher ease of communication; and other diet with higher mobility. Phenotype differences were observed in mobility and communication subdomains.

Table 3. (**A**). Associations between diet and QoL subdomains, in RRMS and ProgMS. (**B**). Associations between wellness activities and QoL subdomains, in RRMS and ProgMS. (**C**). Associations between supplement use, physical activity and QoL subdomains, in RRMS and ProgMS.

(A)

Diet	Anti-Inflammatory		Low Carbohydrate		Low-Saturated Fat		Other	
QoL	RRMS	ProgMS	RRMS	ProgMS	RRMS	ProgMS	RRMS	ProgMS
Physical								
Mobility	−0.09 (−0.97, 0.79)	1.51 (0.17, 2.84) *	−0.34 (−1.35, 0.67)	−0.77 (−0.73, 2.28)	0.10 (−0.97, 1.18)	0.62 (−1.09, 2.34)	−0.64 (−1.56, 0.27)	1.42 (0.07, 2.78) *
Fine motor	−1.06 (−2.26, 0.14)	0.69 (−1.12, 2.50)	−1.09 (−2.47, 0.28)	−0.84 (−2.87, 1.19)	0.35 (−1.11, 1.81)	1.42 (−0.90, 3.74)	−1.24 (−2.50, −0.01)	−0.20 (−2.05, 1.64)
Fatigue	−0.28 (−1.57, 1.00)	−0.02 (−1.96, 1.92)	0.83 (−0.64, 2.30)	−0.93 (−3.11, 1.24)	0.59 (−0.97, 2.15)	−1.53 (−4.01, 0.95)	1.02 (−0.31, 2.34)	−1.51 (−3.48, 0.47)
Sleep disturbance	0.41 (−0.81, 1.64)	0.38 (−1.47, 2.23)	−0.16 (−1.56, 1.24)	0.92 (−1.15, 2.99)	0.15 (−1.33, 1.64)	0.00 (−2.36, 2.37)	0.16 (−0.21, 2.32)	1.01 (−0.87, 2.89)
Mental								
Anxiety	0.08 (−1.11, 1.29)	−0.01 (−1.81, 1.80)	0.03 (−1.34, 1.40)	−0.50 (−2.53, 1.53)	0.89 (−0.56, 2.34)	1.36 (−0.94, 3.65)	0.69 (−0.55, 1.93)	0.08 (−1.76, 1.93)
Depression	0.24 (−0.94, 1.42)	−1.08 (−2.85, 0.70)	−0.11 (−1.46, 1.24)	−1.31 (−3.31, 0.68)	0.38 (−1.05, 1.81)	1.50 (−0.75, 3.76)	1.03 (−0.19, 2.25)	−0.72 (−2.53, 1.09)
Positive affect	0.45 (−0.73, 1.63)	2.05 (0.27, 3.83)	0.54 (−0.81, 1.88)	2.22 (0.23, 4.21)	0.14 (−1.29, 1.57)	−0.03 (−2.31, 2.25)	−0.17 (−1.39, 1.05)	1.55 (−0.27, 3.36)
Emotional dyscontrol	0.51 (−0.87, 1.91)	−0.08 (−2.17, 2.02)	0.20 (−1.38, 1.79)	−1.73 (−4.08, 0.62)	0.63 (−1.05, 2.32)	−0.28 (−2.97, 2.40)	0.91 (−0.53, 2.34)	−0.00 (−2.14, 2.13)
Stigma	1.26 (0.22, 2.30)	−0.12 (−1.68, 1.44)	1.23 (0.04, 2.41)	0.38 (−1.37, 2.13)	0.55 (−0.71, 1.80)	0.25 (−1.76, 2.25)	1.36 (0.29, 2.43)	−0.08 (−1.68, 1.52)
Cognitive function	−0.77 (−2.27, 0.72)	−0.32 (−2.58, 1.94)	−1.04 (−2.75, 0.67)	0.23 (−2.30, 2.77)	−1.04 (−2.85, 0.77)	1.64 (−1.25, 4.53)	−1.92 (−3.46, −0.37)	0.50 (−1.80, 2.79)
Communication [a]	−0.20 (−0.68, 0.29)	0.07 (−0.66, 0.80)	−0.03 (−0.58, 0.52)	−0.06 (−0.88, 0.76)	−0.30 (−0.88, 0.29)	0.00 (−2.36, 2.37)	−0.48 (−0.98, 0.02)	0.26 (−0.48, 1.00)
Social								
Participation	0.27 (−0.73, 1.27)	−0.00 (−1.51, 1.51)	−0.49 (−1.63, 0.66)	−0.28 (−1.98, 1.42)	−0.53 (−1.75, 0.69)	0.38 (−1.54, 2.31)	−1.04 (−2.07, 0.01)	0.50 (−1.03, 2.04)
Satisfaction	0.28 (−0.62, 1.18)	0.77 (−0.59, 2.13)	−0.27 (−1.29, 0.76)	0.05 (−1.48, 1.57)	0.15 (−0.95, 1.24)	0.58 (−1.16, 2.33)	−0.20 (−1.13, 0.73)	0.51 (−0.87, 1.90)

(B)

Wellness	Mind		Mind–Body		Other	
QoL	RRMS	ProgMS	RRMS	ProgMS	RRMS	ProgMS
Physical						
Mobility	−0.82 (−1.71, 0.07)	0.29 (−1.02, 1.61)	0.20 (−0.69, 1.09)	0.95 (−0.34, 2.24)	−0.89 (−1.80, 0.03)	0.48 (−0.81, 1.78)
Fine motor	−1.70 (−2.90, −0.49)	0.09 (−1.68, 1.86)	−0.34 (−1.54, 0.87)	0.57 (−1.18, 2.32)	−1.75 (−2.99, −0.51)	0.64 (−1.11, 2.39) *
Fatigue	1.39 (0.10, 2.68)	1.26 (−0.64, 3.16)	−0.83 (−2.12, 0.45)	−1.46 (−3.33, 0.41)	2.35 (1.03, 3.68)	0.85 (−1.03, 2.72)
Sleep disturbance	1.09 (−0.13, 2.31)	1.72 (−0.09, 3.53)	−1.16 (−2.38, 0.07)	−0.31 (−2.09, 1.47)	1.72 (0.46, 2.99)	0.57 (−1.22, 2.34)
Mental						
Anxiety	2.30 (1.10, 3.49)	1.57 (−0.20, 3.33)	−1.00 (−2.20, 0.20)	−0.62 (−2.36, 1.12)	1.87 (0.63, 3.11)	0.42 (−1.32, 2.16)
Depression	0.95 (−0.23, 2.13)	1.28 (−0.46, 3.02)	−1.06 (−2.24, 0.12)	−0.39 (−0.22, 3.20)	0.92 (−0.30, 2.14)	0.23 (−1.49, 1.95)
Positive affect	−0.40 (−1.58, 0.78)	−0.73 (−2.48, 1.02)	1.44 (0.27, 2.62)	1.49 (−0.22, 3.20)	−0.56 (−1.80, 0.66)	0.11 (−1.61, 1.84)
Emotional dyscontrol	2.03 (0.64, 3.42)	1.58 (−0.47, 3.63)	−1.63 (−3.02, −0.25)	0.50 (−1.51, 2.52)	2.16 (0.72, 3.59)	1.16 (−0.87, 3.17)
Stigma	1.04 (0.01, 2.08)	0.86 (−0.68, 2.40)	0.15 (−0.89, 1.19)	−0.40 (−1.91, 1.11)	1.11 (0.04, 2.19)	0.23 (−1.29, 1.75)
Cognitive function	−1.67 (−3.16, −1.17)	−1.38 (−3.59, 0.84)	0.76 (−0.74, 2.26)	0.26 (−1.92, 2.43)	−3.20 (−4.74, −1.67)	−0.89 (−3.06, 1.28)
Communication [a]	−0.53 (−1.01, −0.05)	−0.42 (−1.13, 0.29)	0.01 (−0.47, 0.50)	0.12 (−0.58, 0.82)	−0.56 (−1.06, −0.07)	−0.39 (−1.10, 0.31)

Table 3. Cont.

(B)

	Wellness		Mind		Mind–Body		Other	
	QoL							
			RRMS	ProgMS	RRMS	ProgMS	RRMS	ProgMS
Social Participation			−1.29 (−2.29, −0.28)	−0.89 (−2.37, 0.59)	1.29 (0.29, 2.29)	1.26 (−0.20, 2.71)	−1.52 (−2.55, −0.49)	−0.99 (−2.45, 0.47)
Satisfaction			−0.99 (−1.90, −0.09)	−0.62 (−1.95, 0.71)	0.83 (−0.08, 1.72)	1.11 (−0.20, 2.42)	−1.24 (−2.18, −0.31)	−0.48 (−1.80, 0.83)

(C)

	Supplements				Physical Activity			
	Vitamin D		Omega-3		Moderate		Active	
	RRMS	ProgMS	RRMS	ProgMS	RRMS	ProgMS	RRMS	ProgMS
QoL								
Physical								
Mobility	0.01 (−1.22, 1.24)	0.40 (−1.20, 2.01)	0.35 (−0.52, 1.25)	0.33 (−0.94, 1.60)	**1.41 (0.19, 2.63)**	−0.31 (−1.88, 1.25)	**3.07 (2.04, 4.09)**	**1.49 (0.05, 2.94)**
Fine motor	−0.39 (−2.05, 1.28)	1.80 (−0.37, 3.97)	−0.34 (−1.54, 0.86)	0.76 (−0.96, 2.47)	0.93 (−0.74, 2.61)	−0.77 (−2.92, 1.38)	**2.45 (1.05, 3.86)**	−0.71 (−2.70, 1.27) *
Fatigue	−1.57 (−3.35, 0.21)	−0.92 (−3.24, 1.41)	−0.61 (−1.90, 0.67)	−0.91 (−2.75, 0.92)	−1.48 (−3.25, 0.29)	−1.35 (−3.63, 0.93)	**−4.14 (−5.63, −2.65)**	**−2.11 (−4.21, −0.01)**
Sleep disturbance	−0.52 (−2.22, 1.17)	−0.52 (−2.73, 1.70)	−0.39 (−1.61, 0.83)	−0.74 (−2.49, 1.01)	−1.20 (−2.91, 0.51)	−1.64 (−3.84, 0.55)	**−2.37 (−3.80, −0.94)**	−1.54 (−3.56, 0.48)
Mental								
Anxiety	0.12 (−1.53, 1.79)	−1.05 (−3.22, 1.12)	0.39 (−0.89, 1.50)	−0.48 (−2.19, 1.23)	**−1.97 (−3.64, −0.31)**	−1.66 (−3.79, 0.48)	**−2.92 (−4.32, −1.52)**	0.37 (−1.60, 2.34) *
Depression	−0.42 (−2.05, 1.22)	−0.28 (−2.41, 1.85)	0.38 (−0.80, 1.55)	0.05 (−1.63, 1.73)	**−2.02 (−3.65, −0.39)**	−1.47 (−3.56, 0.62)	**−3.67 (−5.04, −2.30)**	−0.50 (−2.43, 1.43) *
Positive affect	0.37 (−1.26, 2.01)	−0.82 (−2.95, 1.31)	−0.09 (−1.26, 1.09)	−0.05 (−1.74, 1.63)	**2.51 (0.89, 4.13)**	**2.61 (0.52, 4.69)**	**4.35 (2.99, 5.71)**	0.59 (−1.32, 2.50) *
Emotional dyscontrol	−0.28 (−2.20, 1.65)	−1.09 (−3.60, 1.42)	0.43 (−0.95, 1.82)	0.30 (−1.68, 2.28)	−1.27 (−3.41, 0.66)	−2.15 (−4.63, 0.33)	**−3.11 (−4.73, −1.49)**	0.05 (−2.23, 2.24) *
Stigma	−0.61 (−2.05, 0.83)	−1.28 (−3.15, 0.60)	0.41 (−0.61, 1.45)	−0.23 (−1.71, 1.25)	**−2.30 (−3.73, −0.86)**	−1.51 (−3.36, 0.33)	**−3.11 (−4.32, −1.90)**	−0.30 (−2.01, 1.40) *
Cognitive function	1.15 (−0.92, 3.23)	2.00 (−0.70, 4.70)	−0.07 (−1.56, 1.42)	1.39 (−0.75, 3.52)	1.49 (−0.60, 3.57)	**3.17 (0.50, 5.85)**	**2.85 (1.10, 4.60)**	1.11 (−1.37, 3.57)
Communication[a]	0.12 (−0.56, 0.78)	0.73 (−0.14, 1.60)	−0.28 (−0.76, 0.20)	0.42 (−0.26, 1.11)	0.37 (−0.30, 1.04)	0.93 (0.07, 1.79)	**0.80 (0.23, 1.36)**	0.30 (−0.49, 1.10)
Social								
Social participation	0.69 (−0.70, 2.08)	0.82 (−1.00, 2.63)	−0.06 (−1.06, 0.94)	0.44 (−0.99, 1.87)	1.29 (−0.10, 2.70)	0.95 (−0.83, 2.74)	**2.97 (1.81, 4.14)**	0.80 (−0.84, 2.45) *
Social satisfaction	1.01 (−0.24, 2.26)	0.32 (−1.31, 1.95)	0.73 (−0.16, 1.64)	0.10 (−1.19, 1.39)	**1.64 (0.41, 2.89)**	1.49 (−0.09, 3.08)	**3.71 (2.67, 4.75)**	1.20 (−0.25, 2.66) *

ProgMS = progressive MS; QoL = quality of life; RRMS = relapsing-remitted MS; [a] Total raw score. Multivariate linear regression estimating adjusted regression coefficients (95% CI). Models adjusted for age, sex, BMI, education, disability, and duration since MS diagnosis. Bold values in (A) indicate significant ($p < 0.05$) associations between diet and QoL domains. Bold values in (B) indicate significant ($p < 0.05$) associations between wellness and QoL domains. Bold values in (C) indicate significant ($p < 0.05$) associations between physical activity and QoL subdomains. * Significant (* $p < 0.05$) difference between RRMS and ProgMS.

Wellness activities were associated with physical, mental, and social QoL (Table 3B). In RRMS, mind activities were associated with lower fine motor, cognitive function, communication, social participation, and social satisfaction, and with higher fatigue, anxiety, emotional dyscontrol, and stigma. Mind-body activities were associated with higher positive affect and social participation, and lower emotional dyscontrol. Other wellness activities were associated with lower physical, mental, and social QoL in 10 of 13 subdomains, excepting mobility, depression, and positive affect. No significant associations were observed between wellness activities and QoL in ProgMS. Phenotype differences were only observed between other wellness activities and the fine motor subdomain.

Physical activity was associated with physical, mental, and social QoL (Table 3C). In RRMS, physical activity was dose-dependently associated with higher mobility, positive affect, and social satisfaction; and with lower anxiety, depression, and stigma. Active level of physical activity was additionally associated with higher fine motor, cognitive function, communication, social participation, and lower fatigue, sleep disturbance, and emotional dyscontrol. In ProgMS, moderate physical activity was associated with higher positive affect, cognitive function, and lower communication; and active physical activity with higher mobility and lower fatigue. Phenotype differences were observed in 8 of 13 QoL subdomains.

Neither vitamin D nor omega-3 supplements use were associated with QoL (Table 3C).

4. Discussion

Lifestyle behaviors are known to be associated with QoL in pwMS. To inform potential lifestyle management strategies based on disease course, we assessed associations between diet, vitamin D and omega 3 supplementation, and participation in wellness and physical activities on QoL in pwMS, and whether these associations differed in nature and magnitude between MS phenotypes.

Compared to RRMS, people with ProgMS were older, less likely to be in paid employment, had longer disease duration and greater disability, and had a lower female/male ratio, consistent with previous reports [16,17]. Of lifestyle behaviors assessed, physical activity and QoL differed by phenotype. People with ProgMS were less physically active and had lower QoL in specific physical, mental, and social QoL subdomains, also consistent with prior studies [18,23], and expected given advanced disease stage and greater severity of symptoms adversely affecting QoL, and being likely barriers to performing daily activities and independent living.

High quality, anti-inflammatory, and MS-specific diets have been associated with better mental and physical QoL [5,6]. Our results were mixed and not always aligned with previously reported findings. We identified associations of four diet categories with mental and physical, but not social QoL domains. In RRMS, three of four diet categories were associated with higher stigma, a measure of perceived prejudice and discrimination because of disease, potentially reflective of people who feel greater stigmatisation being more inclined to make changes in their diet in attempt to improve or moderate their condition, or the stigma of adhering to dietary restrictions. Unexpectedly, no positive associations of diet with QoL in RRMS were found; the other diet category, comprising organic, low sodium/sugar and semi-vegetarian diets, was associated with both lower cognitive function and fine motor subdomain scores. Timing of adoption as well as duration and adherence of dietary modification may account for these observations.

In ProgMS, diet was associated with positive affect and ease of communication, perhaps indicative of higher mastery and self-control over MS management. Both anti-inflammatory and other diets were associated with improved mobility, consistent with proposed neuroinflammatory and microbiota-gut-brain-axis disease mechanisms. Though studies have reported associations between diet quality and MS-specific diets with lower depression and fatigue respectively [24,25], we did not observe associations in these symptom subdomains. Discrepancies may be attributable to outcome measure tools in addition to potential additive benefits of adhering to multiple lifestyle behaviors. Phenotype differences were evident only in mobility and communication subdomains. The positive association with mobility in ProgMS, an indicator of disease progression and key contributor to reduced QoL, suggests duration of dietary modification may be a factor, although our data do not allow us to make this conclusion.

No associations between vitamin D or omega-3 supplementation and QoL were observed. Prior studies report mixed evidence for a role of vitamin D supplementation on QoL, with positive associations apparent in pwMS with deficiencies or with an intake of more than 5000 IU/day in addition to sufficient sun-exposure [8,9,26]. Similarly, discrepancies between our observations and that reported for omega-3 and QoL [10], may reflect dose and source of omega-3, or dietary balance of omega-3 and -6. Baseline vitamin and mineral levels, or daily dose, frequency, and duration of supplement use were not captured in the current study.

Participation in wellness activities was associated with physical, mental, and social QoL only for people with RRMS. Mind-body activities, encompassing yoga, Tai Chi, Qigong, and exercise therapy, were associated with positive affect, emotional dyscontrol, and social participation, consistent with past reports of favourable effects of exercise therapy and Tai Chi on mental QoL [12,14]. The non-significant and negative associations observed with mind and other wellness activities with QoL subdomains, some contrary to previously reported [27], may be attributable to category inclusions, adherence to behavior, and/or non-specific symptom assessment. Alternatively, it may be that interactive group wellness activities having positive social interactions may be better interventions for improved mental and social QoL. Phenotype difference was only observed with other wellness and fine motor subdomains. Further investigation capturing information regarding adherence to lifestyle behaviors may provide better insight and is necessary to inform practice recommendations.

The benefits of physical activity on overall health are established [15,28] and supported by our data. We found dose-dependent associations in mobility, social satisfaction, and four mental subdomains in RRMS. Active levels of physical activity were positively associated across 13 QoL subdomains. That common symptoms of fatigue, mobility, anxiety, depression, and cognitive function also showed significant positive associations, highlights the potential value of incorporating regular physical activity in MS management. In people with ProgMS, moderate activity had positive associations for positive affect and cognitive function, and active levels for mobility and fatigue, also encouraging for symptom management through adoption of physical activity. The magnitude of associations was generally stronger in RRMS, especially in active levels. Significant phenotype differences were noted in fine motor, five of seven mental and both social subdomains, suggesting that physical interventions may be best implemented early in disease course, adapted to disease progression.

The strengths of our study are the inclusion of a large and diverse population of pwMS, with minimal participant bias due to the open nature of recruitment, enabling generalizability of findings. Moreover, the large number of participants of RRMS and ProgMS phenotype meant that separation based on disease stage was possible; most prior studies report on mixed phenotype populations. The dataset captures a breadth of clinical and lifestyle variables, enabling robust analysis of associations among a spectrum of behaviors and QoL.

Limitations include self-reported optional survey responses which impact data quality and missingness, and potential selection bias with only 35% participant inclusion for which we controlled by assessing biases between included and excluded participants and adjusting for variables that were significantly different (data not shown). Some participant biases, such as possible increased motivation of pwMS who completed all surveys, are unable to be adjusted for. The cross-sectional analysis limits the inference of causal relationships but provides insight to guide future longitudinal studies. Other factors including socioeconomics, access to health services, and support networks, may also contribute to QoL and should be considered in interpretation of the findings. The use of non-validated tools to capture lifestyle and health outcome variables limits interpretation and comparison with previously reported studies; however, the survey was developed by the multi-stakeholder iConquerMS Research Committee, comprising MS specialist health professionals and scientists, and pwMS, therefore results should be considered alongside other research for practice translation in pwMS. The non-exclusive lifestyle option selections, lack of capture of duration and adherence to behaviors, as well as researcher-defined broad re-categorizations, potentially masked associations; these and other recommendations are being considered for ongoing data capture.

5. Conclusions

Our study demonstrated that lifestyle behaviors concerning diet, wellness, and particularly physical activity, but not vitamin D or omega-3 intake, have positive associations with specific QoL subdomains in pwMS. Some differences in associations between RRMS and ProgMS phenotypes were observed, suggesting a need for phenotype-specific recommendations for MS management. Our findings suggest a role for modifiable lifestyle behaviors as a potential intervention for improving QoL in pwMS. Replication and validation through prospective studies are required to make specific recommendations; however, the presence and absence of associations by phenotype found in our study suggest areas that may be most rewarding for study among certain subgroups.

Author Contributions: Conceptualization, N.N.; methodology, N.N., M.Y.; formal analysis, M.Y.; investigation, H.K.S.; resources, H.K.S., S.L.N.; data curation, M.Y.; writing—original draft preparation, N.N., M.Y.; writing—review and editing, N.N., M.Y., G.A.J., S.S.-Y., S.L.N., H.K.S.; visualization, N.N.; supervision, N.N.; project administration, N.N.; funding acquisition, H.K.S., G.A.J. All authors have read and agreed to the published version of the manuscript.

Funding: Data collection and curation was funded by the Patient-Centered Outcomes Research Institute. Data access and research activity was funded by philanthropic gifts to the Neuroepidemiology Unit from Mr Wal Pisciotta and anonymous donors. Open access fee was funded by Accelerated Cure Project for Multiple Sclerosis.

Institutional Review Board Statement: This study was approved by The University of Melbourne, Melbourne School of Population and Global Health Human Ethics Advisory Group, project #1956113.1.

Informed Consent Statement: Written informed consent has been obtained from all participants.

Data Availability Statement: Restrictions apply to the availability of these data. Data was obtained from Accelerated Cure Project for Multiple Sclerosis and may be requested from HS with the approval of the iConquerMS Research Committee.

Acknowledgments: The authors gratefully acknowledge survey participants, and data collectors and curators of iConquerMS.

Conflicts of Interest: The authors declare no conflict of interest. The funders had no role in the design of the study; in the collection, analyses, or interpretation of data; in the writing of the manuscript, or in the decision to publish the results.

References

1. McGinley, M.P.; Goldschmidt, C.H.; Rae-Grant, A.D. Diagnosis and treatment of multiple sclerosis: A review. *JAMA* **2021**, *325*, 765–779. [CrossRef]
2. Brownlee, W.J.; Hardy, T.A.; Fazekas, F.; Miller, D.H. Diagnosis of multiple sclerosis: Progress and challenges. *Lancet* **2017**, *389*, 1336–1346. [CrossRef]
3. Lublin, F.D.; Reingold, S.C.; Cohen, J.A.; Cutter, G.R.; Sørensen, P.S.; Thompson, A.J.; Wolinsky, J.S.; Balcer, L.J.; Banwell, B.; Barkhof, F. Defining the clinical course of multiple sclerosis: The 2013 revisions. *Neurol. Clin. Neurophysiol.* **2014**, *83*, 278–286. [CrossRef] [PubMed]
4. Gil-González, I.; Martín-Rodríguez, A.; Conrad, R.; Pérez-San-Gregorio, M.Á. Quality of life in adults with multiple sclerosis: A systematic review. *BMJ Open* **2020**, *10*, e041249. [CrossRef] [PubMed]
5. Evers, I.; Heerings, M.; de Roos, N.M.; Jongen, P.J.; Visser, L.H. Adherence to dietary guidelines is associated with better physical and mental quality of life: Results from a cross-sectional survey among 728 dutch ms patients. *Nutr. Neurosci.* **2021**, *2021*, 1–8. [CrossRef]

6. Mousavi-Shirazi-Fard, Z.; Mazloom, Z.; Izadi, S.; Fararouei, M. The effects of modified anti-inflammatory diet on fatigue, quality of life, and inflammatory biomarkers in relapsing-remitting multiple sclerosis patients: A randomized clinical trial. *Int. J. Neurosci.* **2021**, *131*, 657–665. [CrossRef]
7. Hadgkiss, E.J.; Jelinek, G.A.; Weiland, T.J.; Pereira, N.G.; Marck, C.H.; van der Meer, D.M. The association of diet with quality of life, disability, and relapse rate in an international sample of people with multiple sclerosis. *Nutr. Neurosci.* **2015**, *18*, 125–136. [CrossRef] [PubMed]
8. Beckmann, Y.; Türe, S.; Duman, S.U. Vitamin d deficiency and its association with fatigue and quality of life in multiple sclerosis patients. *EPMA J.* **2020**, *11*, 65–72. [CrossRef] [PubMed]
9. Simpson-Yap, S.; Jelinek, P.; Weiland, T.; Nag, N.; Neate, S.; Jelinek, G. Self-reported use of vitamin d supplements is associated with higher physical quality of life scores in multiple sclerosis. *Mult. Scler. Relat. Disord.* **2021**, *49*, 102760. [CrossRef]
10. Jelinek, G.A.; Hadgkiss, E.J.; Weiland, T.J.; Pereira, N.G.; Marck, C.H.; van der Meer, D.M. Association of fish consumption and ω 3 supplementation with quality of life, disability and disease activity in an international cohort of people with multiple sclerosis. *Int. J. Neurosci.* **2013**, *123*, 792–800. [CrossRef]
11. Simpson, R.; Booth, J.; Lawrence, M.; Byrne, S.; Mair, F.; Mercer, S. Mindfulness based interventions in multiple sclerosis-a systematic review. *BMC Neurol.* **2014**, *14*, 1–9. [CrossRef]
12. Taylor, E.; Taylor-Piliae, R.E. The effects of tai chi on physical and psychosocial function among persons with multiple sclerosis: A systematic review. *Complementary Ther. Med.* **2017**, *31*, 100–108. [CrossRef] [PubMed]
13. Benito-Villalvilla, D.; de Uralde-Villanueva, L.; Ríos-León, M.; Álvarez-Melcón, A.C.; Martín-Casas, P. Effectiveness of motor imagery in patients with multiple sclerosis: A systematic review. *Rev. Neurol.* **2021**, *72*, 157–167. [PubMed]
14. Ghahfarrokhi, M.M.; Banitalebi, E.; Negaresh, R.; Motl, R.W. Home-based exercise training in multiple sclerosis: A systematic review with implications for future research. *Mult. Scler. Relat. Disord.* **2021**, *55*, 103177. [CrossRef] [PubMed]
15. Alphonsus, K.B.; Su, Y.; D'Arcy, C. The effect of exercise, yoga and physiotherapy on the quality of life of people with multiple sclerosis: Systematic review and meta-analysis. *Complementary Ther. Med.* **2019**, *43*, 188–195. [CrossRef] [PubMed]
16. Gross, H.J.; Watson, C. Characteristics, burden of illness, and physical functioning of patients with relapsing-remitting and secondary progressive multiple sclerosis: A cross-sectional us survey. *Neuropsychiatr. Dis. Treat.* **2017**, *13*, 1349. [CrossRef] [PubMed]
17. Rooney, S.; Wood, L.; Moffat, F.; Paul, L. Prevalence of fatigue and its association with clinical features in progressive and non-progressive forms of multiple sclerosis. *Mult. Scler. Relat. Disord.* **2019**, *28*, 276–282. [CrossRef]
18. Zhang, W.; Becker, H.; Stuifbergen, A. Comparing health promotion and quality of life in people with progressive versus nonprogressive multiple sclerosis. *Int. J. MS Care* **2020**, *22*, 239–246. [CrossRef]
19. WHO. Body Mass Index. Available online: https://www.euro.who.int/en/health-topics/disease-prevention/nutrition/a-healthy-lifestyle/body-mass-index-bmi (accessed on 10 December 2020).
20. Hohol, M.; Orav, E.; Weiner, H. Disease steps in multiple sclerosis: A simple approach to evaluate disease progression. *Neurol. Clin. Neurophysiol.* **1995**, *45*, 251–255. [CrossRef]
21. Amireault, S.; Godin, G. The godin-shephard leisure-time physical activity questionnaire: Validity evidence supporting its use for classifying healthy adults into active and insufficiently active categories. *Percept. Mot. Ski.* **2015**, *120*, 604–622. [CrossRef]
22. Cella, D.; Lai, J.-S.; Nowinski, C.; Victorson, D.; Peterman, A.; Miller, D.; Bethoux, F.; Heinemann, A.; Rubin, S.; Cavazos, J. Neuroqol: Brief measures of health-related quality of life for clinical research in neurology. *Neurology* **2012**, *78*, 1860–1867. [CrossRef]
23. Rezapour, A.; Kia, A.A.; Goodarzi, S.; Hasoumi, M.; Motlagh, S.N.; Vahedi, S. The impact of disease characteristics on multiple sclerosis patients' quality of life. *Epidemiol. Health* **2017**, *39*, e2017008. [CrossRef] [PubMed]
24. Taylor, K.L.; Simpson, S., Jr.; Jelinek, G.A.; Neate, S.L.; De Livera, A.M.; Brown, C.R.; O'Kearney, E.; Marck, C.H.; Weiland, T.J. Longitudinal associations of modifiable lifestyle factors with positive depression-screen over 2.5-years in an international cohort of people living with multiple sclerosis. *Front. Psychiatry* **2018**, *9*, 526. [CrossRef] [PubMed]
25. Wahls, T.L.; Titcomb, T.J.; Bisht, B.; Eyck, P.T.; Rubenstein, L.M.; Carr, L.J.; Darling, W.G.; Hoth, K.F.; Kamholz, J.; Snetselaar, L.G. Impact of the swank and wahls elimination dietary interventions on fatigue and quality of life in relapsing-remitting multiple sclerosis: The waves randomized parallel-arm clinical trial. *Mult. Scler. J.–Exp. Transl. Clin.* **2021**, *7*, 5399. [CrossRef] [PubMed]
26. Jagannath, V.A.; Filippini, G.; Di Pietrantonj, C.; Asokan, G.V.; Robak, E.W.; Whamond, L.; Robinson, S.A. Vitamin d for the management of multiple sclerosis. *Cochrane Database Syst. Rev.* **2018**, *9*, CD008422. [CrossRef] [PubMed]
27. Shohani, M.; Kazemi, F.; Rahmati, S.; Azami, M. The effect of yoga on the quality of life and fatigue in patients with multiple sclerosis: A systematic review and meta-analysis of randomized clinical trials. *Complementary Ther. Clin. Pract.* **2020**, *39*, 101087. [CrossRef]
28. Dauwan, M.; Begemann, M.J.; Slot, M.I.; Lee, E.H.; Scheltens, P.; Sommer, I.E. Physical exercise improves quality of life, depressive symptoms, and cognition across chronic brain disorders: A transdiagnostic systematic review and meta-analysis of randomized controlled trials. *J. Neuron.* **2021**, *268*, 1222–1246. [CrossRef] [PubMed]

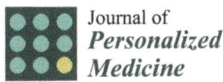

Article

Innovating Care in Multiple Sclerosis: Feasibility of Synchronous Internet-Based Teleconsultation for Longitudinal Clinical Monitoring

Nima Sadeghi [1,2], Piet Eelen [2], Guy Nagels [1,3,4,5], Corinne Cuvelier [2], Katinka Van Gils [2], Marie B. D'hooghe [1,2,3], Jeroen Van Schependom [3,6,†] and Miguel D'haeseleer [1,2,3,*,†]

1. Department of Neurology, Universitair Ziekenhuis Brussel (UZ Brussel), Laarbeeklaan 101, 1090 Brussels, Belgium; nima.sadeghi@uzbrussel.be (N.S.); guy.nagels@uzbrussel.be (G.N.); marie.dhooghe@mscenter.be (M.B.D.)
2. Nationaal Multiple Sclerose Centrum, Vanheylenstraat 16, 1820 Melsbroek, Belgium; piet.eelen@mscenter.be (P.E.); corinne.cuvelier@mscenter.be (C.C.); katinka.vangils@mscenter.be (K.V.G.)
3. Center for Neurosciences (C4N), NEUR and AIMS, Vrije Universiteit Brussel (VUB), Laarbeeklaan 103, 1090 Brussels, Belgium; jeroen.van.schependom@vub.be
4. Icometrix, Kolonel Begaultlaan 1b, 3012 Leuven, Belgium
5. Zebra Academy, Researchdreef 12, 1070 Brussels, Belgium
6. Department of Electronics and Informatics (ETRO), Vrije Universiteit Brussel (VUB), Pleinlaan 2, 1050 Brussels, Belgium
* Correspondence: miguel.dhaeseleer@uzbrussel.be; Tel.: +32-2-477-60-12
† These authors contributed equally to this work.

Abstract: The 'coronavirus disease of 2019' crisis has recently forced an expedited adoption of teleconsultation (TC) in most medical domains. Short-term digital interventions have generally been associated with feasibility, clinical benefits, user satisfaction, and cost-effectiveness in patients with multiple sclerosis (MS) but outcomes after repeated utilization over extended periods need to be further evaluated. In this feasibility study, 60 subjects with MS were 1:1 randomized to receive standard care augmented by four TCs using an audiovisual Internet platform (intervention) versus standard care alone (controls), over a period of 12 months. Effects on functional status, medical costs, and satisfaction were explored as secondary outcomes. Eighty-nine out of 108 scheduled TCs (82.4%) were completed, and 26 patients could complete at least one TC (86.7%), meeting our prespecified feasibility target of 80%. The intervention did not lead to significant differences in functional status (with the potential exception of fatigue) nor medical costs. Most interventional patients declared themselves to be (very) satisfied about the quality of care and technical aspects associated with the TCs. Our results demonstrate that longitudinal clinical monitoring using real-time audiovisual TC over the Internet is feasible and well-received by patients with MS. Such an approach can be a promising new care strategy.

Keywords: multiple sclerosis; teleconsultation; internet; feasibility; digital health

1. Introduction

Modern society, including the way we practice medicine, has been shaped by the technological progress inherited from the three industrial revolutions that have taken place since the mid-eighteenth century. An extension of the third phase is currently unfolding, characterized by a shift towards digital electronics, augmenting computing power, artificial intelligence, and a dominant role for the Internet. Telemedicine (TM)—sometimes also referred to as e-health or digital medicine—can be defined as the exchange of medical information between patients and healthcare providers, who are in separate locations, by means of electronic communication technology [1]. Phone calls and video conferencing are prototypical examples of directly interactive sessions in real-time, whereas their asynchronous counterparts (e.g., texting, email, self-scoring devices, wearable sensors, instructive tools) rely on store-and-forward transmission of medical data and/or advice [2,3]. TM applications have originally been developed to enable medical services that are difficult to deliver face-to-face, mainly due to time-sensitive requirements or geographic hurdles, but are now increasingly and more widely solicited as a complementary support in conjunction with the more traditional customs [4,5]. Especially in 2020, digital medicine has undergone an expedited adoption, as the 'coronavirus disease of 2019' (COVID-19) rapidly evolved into a global crisis, for which unprecedented social isolation and mobility restrictions have been installed as key measures of constrain [6,7], with teleconsultation (TC) becoming an essential escape scenario for a vast proportion of our health system [8–10].

Studies that have explored the impact of TM in patients with multiple sclerosis (MS), a frequently occurring, chronic inflammatory demyelinating and degenerative disorder of the central nervous system [11], were heterogeneous in terms of intervention type, methodology, and objectives (i.e., disability assessment, disease management, remote treatment, rehabilitation/exercise) but have generally shown that the applied procedures provide clinical benefit, user satisfaction, time gain, and/or cost-effectiveness [3,12]. Notably though, scientific data on synchronous communication for TC purposes remain scarce in this field. Two independent pilot studies have recently demonstrated that such single sessions, using an audiovisual Internet platform, were feasible and well-received in patients with MS [13,14]. The outcomes after repeated utilization over extended periods of time, however, are still unknown and form the subject of our current paper, hereby addressing an important and actual knowledge gap in the anticipation that TC—once we have reached the post-COVID-19 era—will consolidate its newly obtained place in the MS clinic [15].

2. Materials and Methods

2.1. Study Design, Objectives and Ethics

We performed a single-center prospective study exploring the feasibility (primary endpoint) of multiple planned synchronous TCs, using an audiovisual Internet platform, in the longitudinal clinical monitoring of patients with MS. Effects on functional status, medical costs estimates, and satisfaction were assessed as secondary outcomes; a randomized control trial design was adopted because most of these exploratory analyses required a comparison to standard care. Our study was approved by the ethics committee of the Nationaal Multiple Sclerose Centrum (NMSC) Melsbroek (local; internal reference: AvN/AVDZ) and the Universitair Ziekenhuis Brussel (leading; internal reference: 2018/269, Belgian Unique Number: 143201836797). Written informed consent was obtained from all participants prior to inclusion. Recruitment and teleconsulting procedures were similar to a preparatory pilot, in which one digital visit was planned in twenty patients with MS [14], who all agreed to be involved in this longitudinal project as well.

2.2. Participants

Sixty French- and/or Dutch-speaking patients with MS, according to the 2017 revised McDonald criteria [16], were recruited at the NMSC Melsbroek, which is a specialized Belgian MS center, during routine medical follow-up. Home access to the Internet with a webcam-equipped device was mandatory for study participation. Inclusion of individuals with a high suspicion of moderate to severe cognitive impairment (based on common sense judgement of the medical record and/or initial patient contact; any known cognitive dysfunction defined as scoring less than 21 on the Mini Mental State Evaluation, if present in the medical record, was used as an exclusion criteria) was actively avoided. Eligible candidates were 1:1 randomized to receive standard care (control group) versus standard care, augmented by four scheduled TM visits (intervention group) over the following 12 months, using "Research Randomizer" (https://randomizer.org; last accessed on 22 February 2020).

2.3. Teleconsultations

The study period started with an inclusion visit and terminated with a close-out evaluation (both face-to-face), conducted by the study supervisor (MiD), with an interval of 12 ± 2 months between both. Subjects in the intervention group received the date and time of their first TC after randomization, and subsequent appointments were planned at the end of each digital contact, striving for an equal distribution over the study period (i.e., one TC every 3 months). The rescheduling of digital appointments was permitted as this regularly occurs with standard visits as well. All TCs were performed by the same MS nurse or neurologist—derived from a pool of three consulting nurses (PE, CC, KVG) and one neurologist (MiD)—for each individual patient, using an Internet-based audiovisual communication platform obtained from Zebra Academy [17]. The main goal of the TCs was to explore the patient's current global health status during a routine clinical consult. A checklist (with questions about e.g., general and neurological health, medication, and life-style factors—see Table in Ref. [14]), similar to the usual content of a regular face-to-face MS consultation, was used as the backbone for the conversation, but deviations at the patient's initiative were allowed. Patients were provided with a unique hyperlink by email in advance, leading them directly to the virtual waiting room where they could see and accept our incoming call (see Figure in Ref. [14]). Access was possible from any device with a webcam (i.e., laptop, desktop, tablet, smartphone). Google Chrome (Google LLC, Mountain View, CA, USA) was used as the web browser on both sides of the connection, as advised by Zebra Academy. All subjects had 30 min to respond to the call, starting from the scheduled time, with maximum of three attempts. A written report was forwarded by the study team to the treating neurologist after each TC.

2.4. Evaluations

2.4.1. Feasibility

Our TC approach was considered feasible if at least 80% of the patients in the intervention group could complete at least one digital visit and if at least 80% of the total number of scheduled digital visits could be completed (a priori defined).

2.4.2. Functional Status

Clinical relapses during the study period were recorded, as self-reported by the patients, at the close-out visit. Disability, clustered symptomatology, and health-related quality of life were assessed at both the inclusion and close-out visit. The following variables were recorded: general disability with the Expanded Disability Status Scale (EDSS), mobility with the Timed 25-Foot Walk Test (T25FWT), dexterity with the Nine-Hole Peg Test (9HPT), information-processing speed with the Symbol Digit Modalities Test (SDMT), fatigue with the Fatigue Severity Scale (FSS), depression with the Beck Depression Inventory (BDI) and the Hospital Anxiety and Depression Scale (HADS), anxiety with the HADS, sleep quality with the Pittsburgh Sleep Quality Index (PSQI), and overall health-related quality of life with the Multiple Sclerosis Impact Scale (MSIS-29).

2.4.3. Medical Costs

The number of emergency room visits, days of hospital admission (not including the study site) and visits to the general practitioner over the study period, as self-reported by the patients, were recorded at the close-out visit, as a proxy of medical costs.

2.4.4. Satisfaction

The satisfaction with the study trajectory was enquired about for all patients, and their respective digital caregiver if applicable, at the close-out visit by means of 5-point Likert scales containing the following categories: very unsatisfied, unsatisfied, neutral, satisfied, very satisfied. Assessments were independently carried out for (a) global quality of care, (b) technical quality of the TCs, (c) convenience of the TCs, (d) quality of care of the TCs, and (e) added value of the TCs to medical care. Only item (a) was relevant for participants of the control group. Quantification per item was performed by giving a score of one for responding 'very unsatisfied' and increasing by one point for each higher response category.

2.5. COVID-19 Interference

Patients were enrolled in this project from 26 August 2019 to 21 February 2020. Due to unexpected COVID-19 measures, non-urgent medical appointments had to be postponed in Belgium on multiple occasions during the course of the study (particularly March–June and October–November 2020). This resulted in (a) two close-out evaluations falling outside the foreseen time frame (15 and 16 months after the inclusion visit, respectively) and (b) the need for scheduling several TCs sooner than initially intended. Timelines containing inclusion, close-out and all TC visits for each participant of the intervention group are displayed in the Figure 1.

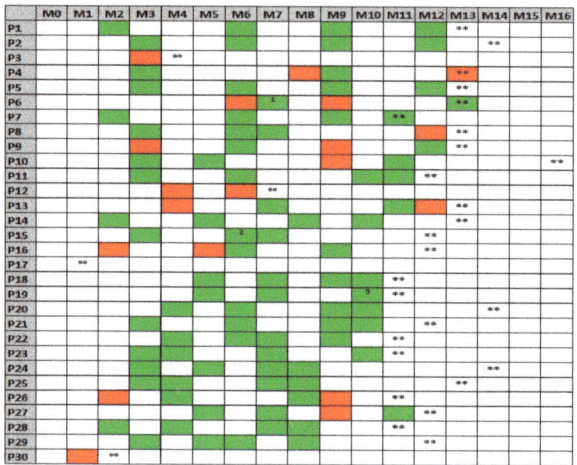

Figure 1. Timeline of study visits for each participant of the intervention group. M: month, P: patient. ** close out visit, °° drop-out. Successful teleconsultations are indicated in green, unsuccessful attempts in red. Corrections: 1 the successful teleconsultation was performed at M6, 2 two successful teleconsultations were performed at M6, 3 two successful teleconsultations were performed at M10.

2.6. Statistics

All statistical procedures were performed with GraphPad Prism version 9.0.0 (GraphPad Software; San Diego, CA, USA). Data are expressed as mean ± SD for reasons of uniformity. Group differences were assessed by means of unpaired Student t tests or Mann–Whitney U tests, where appropriate, depending on the data distribution revealed by Shapiro–Wilk testing. All reported p values are two-tailed and were considered statistically significant at the 0.05 level.

2.7. Data Availability

Anonymized data will be shared upon reasonable request from any qualified investigator.

3. Results

3.1. Participants

Baseline demographical data of all participants are shown in Table 1. Twenty-four of the patients randomized to the intervention group were under disease-modifying treatment at study inclusion (interferon beta: 1; teriflunomide: 1; dimethylfumarate: 3; fingolimod: 1; ocrelizumab: 4; natalizumab: 8; alemtuzumab: 6), versus 26 of the controls (interferon beta: 5; glatiramere acetate: 4; teriflunomide: 3; dimethylfumarate: 3; fingolimod: 1;

ocrelizumab: 4; natalizumab: 6). Four subjects in each group dropped out during the study; reasons were loss of follow-up (one intervention subject who cancelled his first TC versus three controls), loss of interest (two intervention subjects versus one control), and a suitable device being no longer available (one intervention subject). Timing of drop-out in the intervention group can be deduced from the Figure 1.

Table 1. Baseline demographic of the study participants.

	Intervention Group	Control Group
Number of subjects	30	30
Age * [years]	41.3 (10.4)	45.9 (9.1)
Gender [Female/Male]	19/11	15/15
MS subtype [RR/SP/PP]	21/8/1	21/7/2
Disease duration * [years]	10.1 (7.1)	11.2 (6.4)
Education [ES/HS/HE]	0/8/22	3/15/12
Employment status [U/E/S/D/R]	1/14/0/14/1	0/10/1/19/0

MS: multiple sclerosis, RR: relapsing-remitting, SP: secondary progressive, PP: primary progressive, ES: elementary school, HS: high school, HE: higher education, U: unemployed, E: employed (active), S: sick leave (temporary), D: disability leave (permanent), R: retired. * Data expressed as mean (SD).

3.2. Feasibility

Eighty-nine out of 108 scheduled TCs (82.4%) were successfully completed during the study while 26 patients could successfully complete at least one TC (86.7%). Failures were due to patients not responding (14/19) and technical issues (5/19). The non-responders were contacted at a later time by telephone and advised us that they either had forgotten the appointment or did not want to participate any longer (two subjects). Technical issues included no notification of the incoming call (three occasions), difficulties maintaining the Internet connection (one occasion), and insufficient quality of sound (one occasion). Isolated success rates were 21/29 (72.4%) for TC-1, 24/27 (88.9%) for TC-2, and 22/26 (84.6%) for TC-3 and -4.

3.3. Functional Status

The mean number of patient-reported relapses during the study period did not differ between participants of the intervention and control groups (0.3 ± 0.5 each, $p = 0.54$) who completed the study. Results of all other functional outcome measures are shown in Tables 2 and 3. Mean changes were not statistically significant except for the FSS scores, which decreased by 0.3 ± 1.2 in patients of the intervention group, compared with an increase of 0.4 ± 1.0 in those of the control group ($p = 0.03$).

3.4. Medical Costs

No significant differences were observed in the mean number of emergency room visits (0.3 ± 0.5 versus 0.2 ± 0.5, $p = 0.91$), days of hospital admission (0.7 ± 2.7 versus 2.7 ± 8.0, $p = 0.18$), and the number of visits to a general practitioner (3.1 ± 4.5 versus 2.1 ± 2.1, $p = 0.77$) over the study period between patients of the intervention and control groups, respectively, who completed the study.

3.5. Satisfaction

Quantified results of the satisfaction enquiry are demonstrated in Table 4. The proportion of patients in the intervention group—who completed the study—declaring themselves to be satisfied or highly satisfied was 26/26 for global quality of care, 19/26 for technical quality of the TCs, 24/26 for convenience of the TCs, 24/26 for quality of care of the TCs, and 23/26 for added value of the TCs to medical care; results for the health professionals who performed the TCs were 25/26, 16/26, 21/26, 25/26, and 25/26, respectively.

Table 2. Functional outcomes in patients randomized to the intervention group who completed the study (N = 26) *.

	Inclusion	Close-Out	Change
EDSS	4.2 (2.1) [0]	4.2 (2.3) [0]	0.1 (0.9) [0]; 0.82
T25FWT	15.6 (34.4) [0]	26.6 (53.1) [1]	10.8 (34.1) [1]; 0.75
9HPT-dom	25.6 (13.7) [0]	24.7 (9.9) [1]	−0.8 (11.8) [1]; 0.82
9HPT-ndom	34.4 (53.5) [0]	37.4 (55.0) [1]	2.4 (11.9) [1]; 0.77
SDMT	58.3 (12.5) [2]	55.0 (13.6) [2]	−1.8 (10.0) [4]; 0.38
FSS	4.9 (1.2) [0]	4.6 (1.7) [0]	−0.3 (1.2) [0]; 0.03
BDI	10.9 (7.2) [0]	11.5 (11.4) [0]	0.7 (6.9) [0]; 0.56
HADS-anx	6.7 (4.0) [0]	6.3 (4.9) [0]	−0.3 (5.3) [0]; 0.55
HADS-dep	5.0 (3.5) [0]	5.5 (5.2) [0]	0.5 (4.6) [0]; 0.58
PSQI	6.3 (3.7) [1]	6.8 (4.7) [5]	−0.2 (4.0) [5]; 0.69
MSIS-29-phy	29.1 (20.2) [1]	34.6 (24.8) [0]	4.8 (18.1) [1]; 0.33
MSIS-29-psy	29.2 (22.5) [3]	29.2 (24.2) [0]	1.3 (23.9) [3]; 0.79

EDSS: Expanded Disability Status Scale; T25FWT: Timed 25-Foot Walk Test; 9HPT-dom: Nine-Hole Peg Test for dominant hand; 9HPT-ndom: Nine-Hole Peg Test for non-dominant hand; SDMT: Symbol Digit Modalities Test; FSS: Fatigue Severity Scale; BDI: Beck Depression Inventory; HADS-anx: Hospital Anxiety and Depression Scale for anxiety; HADS-dep: Hospital Anxiety and Depression Scale for depression; PSQI: Pittsburgh Sleep Quality Index (PSQI); MSIS-29-psy: Multiple Sclerosis Impact Scale for psychological impact; MSIS-29-phy: Multiple Sclerosis Impact Scale for physical impact. * Scores expressed as mean (SD) [missing values]; p value for comparison with the respective change in the control group, as expressed in Table 3.

Table 3. Functional outcomes in patients randomized to the control group who completed the study (N = 26) *.

	Inclusion	Close-Out	Change
EDSS	4.4 (2.1) [0]	4.6 (2.0) [0]	0.2 (0.7) [0]
T25FWT	6.8 (2.9) [2]	27.9 (74.3) [0]	0.8 (2.2) [2]
9HPT-dom	48.9 (74.0) [0]	54.6 (77.9) [0]	5.6 (20.7) [0]
9HPT-ndom	50.0 (73.7) [0]	52.0 (74.4) [0]	2.1 (6.3) [0]
SDMT	53.6 (14.5) [4]	52.5 (13.9) [1]	0.9 (9.6) [5]
FSS	4.3 (1.2) [0]	4.6 (1.5) [0]	0.4 (1.0) [0]
BDI	8.8 (5.7) [0]	7.4 (4.9) [1]	−1.4 (3.8) [1]
HADS-anx	6.1 (3.6) [0]	6.4 (3.5) [1]	0.4 (3.7) [1]
HADS-dep	4.8 (3.1) [0]	4.5 (2.5) [1]	−0.2 (3.0) [1]
PSQI	6.4 (3.9) [0]	5.8 (3.4) [2]	−0.7 (3.4) [2]
MSIS-29-phy	33.1 (16.2) [3]	39.5 (18.2) [0]	7.7 (11.2) [3]
MSIS-29-psy	29.1 (22.0) [4]	29.8 (17.6) [0]	1.9 (17.6) [4]

EDSS: Expanded Disability Status Scale; T25FWT: Timed 25-Foot Walk Test; 9HPT-dom: Nine-Hole Peg Test for dominant hand; 9HPT-ndom: Nine-Hole Peg Test for non-dominant hand; SDMT: Symbol Digit Modalities Test; FSS: Fatigue Severity Scale; BDI: Beck Depression Inventory; HADS-anx: Hospital Anxiety and Depression Scale for anxiety; HADS-dep: Hospital Anxiety and Depression Scale for depression; PSQI: Pittsburgh Sleep Quality Index (PSQI); MSIS-29-psy: Multiple Sclerosis Impact Scale for psychological impact; MSIS-29-phy: Multiple Sclerosis Impact Scale for physical impact. * Scores expressed as mean (SD) [missing values].

Table 4. Satisfaction as quantified from 5-point Likert scales with regard to patients who completed the study *.

	Intervention Group (N = 26)	Control Group (N = 26)	HCPs Performing the TCs
Global QoC	4.6 (0.5) °	4.5 (0.5) °	4.4 (0.6)
Technical quality of the TCs	4.1 (1.0)	-	3.9 (1.0)
Convenience of the TCs	4.5 (0.6)	-	4.2 (0.9)
QoC of the TCs	4.5 (0.6)	-	4.3 (0.7)
Added value of the TCs to medical care	4.4 (0.7)	-	4.6 (0.6)

HCPs: healthcare providers; TCs: teleconsultations; QoC: quality of care. * Scores expressed as mean (SD); ° p value not significant (0.58).

4. Discussion

We present the first ever study, to our knowledge, demonstrating the feasibility of synchronous TC using an audiovisual Internet platform, when repeatedly applied for the clinical monitoring of individuals with MS over a substantial time period (i.e., one year). In addition, the appraisal of general care, technical quality, and convenience, as related to the digital visits, was excellent in the majority of patients and healthcare providers involved in the interventional arm. These results are in line with a recent and similarly designed trial among subjects with Parkinson disease—representing another frequently occurring chronic disorder of the central nervous system—living throughout the United States of America, in which 98% of the 97 participants randomized to the intervention group completed at least one digital visit, and 91% of the 388 planned digital visits were completed as scheduled. Here, the authors calculated that each virtual session would have saved patients a median of 88 min (95% CI 70–120; $p < 0.001$) and 38 miles per visit (95% CI 36–56; $p < 0.001$), compared to their usual care [18]. Feasibility was considered as a binary outcome measure in both studies (i.e., either the TC works or not) and the prespecified success target of at least 80% corresponds well to previously reported 'no-show' rates associated with in-person visits at neurology clinics [19,20].

Our TC approach did not lead to significant differences in parameters reflecting functional status (with the exception of fatigue) and medical costs. These secondary analyses were incorporated mainly for exploratory purposes, accepting a possible risk of a type II error. The likelihood of inducing a clinically relevant benefit with our intervention was considered low during study preparation, since it was never the intention to offer specific nor standardized treatment programs. Nonetheless, retaining the status quo can also be valuable as we, a priori, did consider the possibility of (increased) virtual attention inducing or aggravating MS-related symptomatology, such as anxiety and/or sleep difficulties. The positive impact of the intervention on fatigue levels should be interpreted with caution because the effect size was small and would not have survived a statistical (Bonferoni) correction for multiple comparisons. It is worth noting, however, that fatigue and physical activity levels showed improvement with other web- and telephone-based interactive sessions primarily based on educational and motivational coaching [21,22]. Surrogates of medical costs did not significantly differ between our two groups and were preferred above direct values because TC still occurred in addition to standard care. Gain in that domain, though, can be expected in future studies which actually replace face-to-face with digital visits in routine follow-up.

COVID-19 has deeply disrupted human socialization and forced our health system towards a large-scale adoption of TC on very short notice. Our findings can help solidify the scientific basis for continuing such practice, using the Internet as the flagship of modern-day communication, within a complementary hybrid model for next-generation MS care [15]. A number of reasons can be given to explain why patients with MS may be particularly suitable candidates to benefit from digitalization of neurological care. First, diagnosis is typically established during young adulthood [11], when time availability for medical attention is limited due to other priorities in life. Second, MS may lead to cumulative physical disability [11], complicating access to neurological facilities, even in areas offering sufficient and dense resources. Third, over the past two decades, we have seen a spectacular growth of the disease-modifying and symptomatic treatment armamentarium for individuals with MS, which is expected to ameliorate at least short- to medium-term prognosis but also increases the complexity of routine follow-up. Fourth, a significant proportion of affected patients (i.e., 30%) appears to completely miss out on neurological care [23], likely decreasing their chance of receiving state-of-the-art disease management and jeopardizing a favorable clinical outcome. Simultaneously, there seems to be a high interest among individuals with MS for using the Internet as a health information source and for online interaction with medical specialists [24]. As a final, general, and perhaps most convincing argument, we can state that nervous system disorders are currently the leading source of disability, affecting over one billion people worldwide [25], and represent a burden that is expected to at least double over the next two decades, mostly because of a growing elderly population [26]. In parallel, we have recently witnessed an increased prevalence and life-expectancy in patients with MS [27,28]. Access to neurological care is indigent already, as expressed by several health authorities in statements that do not solely apply to remote or low-income regions [4]. Consequently, the pressure on our classic health model will naturally rise to levels necessitating at least some form of digital redesign in order to avoid a total overflow, a rationale that has recently been put to the forefront by COVID-19 but survives even in complete abstraction of this crisis.

The most important limitations of this study were caused by the heterogeneity of the healthcare provider pool and the absence of a clinical neurological exam in the TC protocol. Neurology has long remained a very bedside-orientated 'hands-on' specialty, and the fear of missing subtle yet critical clinical details during a remote physical evaluation likely forms the Achilles heel of teleneurology in general. Supportive proposals are starting to be published [3,29], and it is of interest to mention that Bove and colleagues recently reported an agreement within one point between in-person and televideo-enabled EDSS scores for 88% of the cases, which is similar to the in-person inter-rater reliability described earlier by others [30]. The NMSC Melsbroek is a highly specialized hospital specifically focusing on the neurological management, multidisciplinary care, and/or rehabilitation of individuals with MS. All participants were allowed to use the ambulatory and in-hospital rehabilitation services of the center as a part of standard care during the study, if deemed necessary by their treating physicians. This decision was based on ethical considerations, but it cannot be excluded that such rehabilitation activities have influenced our secondary outcomes. As explained above (see Section 3.5), a priori unforeseen COVID-19 measures may have resulted in reduced access to the clinic and/or delay of standard care on multiple occasions during the study, which could have created a disproportionately positive welcoming of digital solutions. Furthermore, there might be other reasons to be cautious when generalizing our findings to the full MS community, as it cannot be ruled out that disease-specific, geographic, cultural, and/or social differences may lead to less positive outcomes. Previous studies have disclosed that patients with cognitive or visual impairment experienced more difficulties while using home-based TM systems [31,32], whereas we have actively avoided recruitment of participants with apparent cognitive dysfunction. We also have to acknowledge that there was a greater proportion of participants with a higher education level in our interventional group, as compared to the controls. TM has generally been praised for its potential to facilitate access to medical care, but recent reports have, somewhat surprisingly, warned of the persistence or even aggravation of ethnical and other disparities [33–35]. Possible solutions include wide-spread promotional campaigns, mobile paramedical teams, assistance by (educated) caregivers, and fully equipped community centers, of which most examples can also help with the more challenging aspects of the clinical exam. These factors related to background variability should not be forgotten when designing future research aimed at demonstrating the non-inferiority of replacing face-to-face with digital visits in the MS clinic, compared to the classic approach.

In conclusion, our study demonstrated the technical and practical feasibility of live audiovisual TC over the Internet for routine neurological follow-up in patients with MS. The digital approach was well-appreciated by both participating patients and healthcare providers. Future trials can now be designed in which the effect (e.g., non-inferiority) of replacing classic face-to-face visits with such TM modalities can be assessed for multiple purposes. We believe that this will be the phase where their full potential will come to expression but also one in which we must factor in the abovementioned systemic pitfalls and tailor the interventions to the individual patient needs.

Author Contributions: M.D. and G.N. conceptualized the study. The statistical analyses were conducted by M.D., G.N. and J.V.S.; N.S. and M.D. wrote the first draft of the paper, while all authors were involved in the critical reading and revision process. All authors have read and agreed to the published version of the manuscript.

Funding: This research received no external competitive funding.

Institutional Review Board Statement: Our study was approved by the ethics committee of the Nationaal Multiple Sclerose Centrum (NMSC) Melsbroek (local; internal reference: AvN/AVDZ) and the Universitair Ziekenhuis Brussel (leading; internal reference: 2018/269, Belgian Unique Number: 143201836797).

Informed Consent Statement: Informed consent was obtained from all subjects involved in the study.

Data Availability Statement: Anonymized data will be shared upon reasonable request from any qualified investigator.

Acknowledgments: The authors thank Zebra Academy for offering their technology free of charge for this study. We would also like to express our gratitude toward Gert Ooms and Ann Van Remoortel (NMSC Nursing Deparment), Thomas Van Oosthuysen (NMSC Information and Communications Technology Department) and the Zebra Academy crew for providing logistic and/or technical support.

Conflicts of Interest: This study was supported by a non-competitive research grant from Roche (Basel, Switzerland). G.N. is a shareholder of Zebra Academy. The authors have no potential conflicts of interest to report.

References

1. Sola-Valls, N.; Blanco, Y.; Sepúlveda, M.; Martinez-Hernandez, E.; Saiz, A. Telemedicine for Monitoring MS Activity and Progression. *Curr. Treat. Options Neurol.* **2015**, *17*, 47. [CrossRef]
2. Rubin, M.N.; Wellik, K.E.; Channer, D.D.; Demaerschalk, B.M. Systematic review of teleneurology: Neurohospitalist neurology. *Neurohospitalist* **2013**, *3*, 120–124. [CrossRef]
3. Xiang, X.M.; Bernard, J. Telehealth in Multiple Sclerosis Clinical Care and Research. *Curr. Neurol. Neurosci. Rep.* **2021**, *21*, 14. [CrossRef] [PubMed]
4. Dorsey, E.R.; Glidden, A.M.; Holloway, M.R.; Birbeck, G.L.; Schwamm, L.H. Teleneurology and mobile technologies: The future of neurological care. *Nat. Rev. Neurol.* **2018**, *14*, 285–297. [CrossRef]
5. Hatcher-Martin, J.M.; Adams, J.L.; Anderson, E.R.; Bove, R.; Burrus, T.M.; Chehrenama, M.; O'Brien, M.D.; Eliashiv, D.S.; Erten-Lyons, D.; Giesser, B.S.; et al. Telemedicine in neurology: Telemedicine Work Group of the American Academy of Neurology update. *Neurology* **2020**, *94*, 30–38. [CrossRef]
6. Rothan, H.A.; Byrareddy, S.N. The epidemiology and pathogenesis of coronavirus disease (COVID-19) outbreak. *J. Autoimmun.* **2020**, *109*, 102433. [CrossRef]
7. Guzik, A.K.; Switzer, J.A. Teleneurology is neurology. *Neurology* **2020**, *94*, 16–17. [CrossRef]
8. Klein, B.C.; Busis, N.A. COVID-19 is catalyzing the adoption of teleneurology. *Neurology* **2020**, *94*, 903–904. [CrossRef] [PubMed]
9. Keesara, S.; Jonas, A.; Schulman, K. Covid-19 and Health Care's Digital Revolution. *N. Engl. J. Med.* **2020**, *382*, e82. [CrossRef]
10. Sastre-Garriga, J.; Tintore, M.; Montalban, X. Keeping standards of multiple sclerosis care through the COVID-19 pandemic. *Mult. Scler.* **2020**, *26*, 1153–1156. [CrossRef]
11. Reich, D.S.; Lucchinetti, C.F.; Calabresi, P.A. Multiple Sclerosis. *N. Engl. J. Med.* **2018**, *378*, 169–180. [CrossRef] [PubMed]
12. Yeroushalmi, S.; Maloni, H.; Costello, K.; Wallin, M.T. Telemedicine and Multiple Sclerosis: A Comprehensive Literature Review. *J. Telemed. Telecare* **2020**, *26*, 400–413. [CrossRef] [PubMed]
13. Robb, J.F.; Hyland, M.H.; Goodman, A.D. Comparison of telemedicine versus in-person visits for persons with multiple sclerosis: A randomized crossover study of feasibility, cost, and satisfaction. *Mult. Scler. Relat. Disord.* **2019**, *36*, 101258. [CrossRef] [PubMed]

14. D'Haeseleer, M.; Eelen, P.; Sadeghi, N.; D'Hooghe, M.B.; Van Schependom, J.; Nagels, G. Feasibility of Real Time Internet-Based Teleconsultation in Patients With Multiple Sclerosis: Interventional Pilot Study. *J. Med. Internet Res.* **2020**, *22*, e18178. [CrossRef] [PubMed]
15. D'Haeseleer, M. Teleconsultation will replace most face-to-face interactions in the multiple sclerosis clinic—Commentary. *Mult. Scler.* **2021**, *27*, 178–179. [CrossRef] [PubMed]
16. Thompson, A.J.; Banwell, B.L.; Barkhof, F.; Carroll, W.M.; Coetzee, T.; Comi, G.; Correale, J.; Fazekas, F.; Filippi, M.; Freedman, M.S.; et al. Diagnosis of multiple sclerosis: 2017 revisions of the McDonald criteria. *Lancet Neurol.* **2018**, *17*, 162–173. [CrossRef]
17. Valenzuela Espinoza, A.; Van Hooff, R.J.; De Smedt, A.; Moens, M.; Yperzeele, L.; Nieboer, K.; Hubloue, I.; de Keyser, J.; Convents, A.; Fernandez Tellez, H.; et al. Development and Pilot Testing of 24/7 In-Ambulance Telemedicine for Acute Stroke: Prehospital Stroke Study at the Universitair Ziekenhuis Brussel-Project. *Cerebrovasc. Dis.* **2016**, *42*, 15–22. [CrossRef] [PubMed]
18. Beck, C.A.; Beran, D.B.; Biglan, K.M.; Boyd, C.M.; Dorsey, E.R.; Schmidt, P.N.; Simone, R.; Willis, A.W.; Galifianakis, N.B.; Katz, M.; et al. National randomized controlled trial of virtual house calls for Parkinson disease. *Neurology* **2017**, *89*, 1152–1161. [CrossRef] [PubMed]
19. Morera-Guitart, J.; Mas-Server, M.A.; Mas-Sese, G. Analysis of the patients who missed their appointments at the neurology clinic of the Marina Alta. *Rev. Neurol.* **2002**, *34*, 701–705. [PubMed]
20. Guzek, L.M.; Gentry, S.D.; Golomb, M.R. The estimated cost of "no-shows" in an academic pediatric neurology clinic. *Pediatr. Neurol.* **2015**, *52*, 198–201. [CrossRef]
21. D'Hooghe, M.; Van Gassen, G.; Kos, D.; Bouquiaux, O.; Cambron, M.; Decoo, D.; Lysandropoulos, A.; van Wijmeersch, B.; Willekens, B.; Penner, I.; et al. Improving fatigue in multiple sclerosis by smartphone-supported energy management: The MS TeleCoach feasibility study. *Mult. Scler. Relat. Disord.* **2018**, *22*, 90–96. [CrossRef] [PubMed]
22. Finlayson, M.; Preissner, K.; Cho, C.; Plow, M. Randomized trial of a teleconference-delivered fatigue management program for people with multiple sclerosis. *Mult. Scler.* **2011**, *17*, 1130–1140. [CrossRef] [PubMed]
23. Minden, S.L.; Hoaglin, D.C.; Hadden, L.; Frankel, D.; Robbins, T.; Perloff, J. Access to and utilization of neurologists by people with multiple sclerosis. *Neurology* **2008**, *70*, 1141–1149. [CrossRef]
24. Lejbkowicz, I.; Paperna, T.; Stein, N.; Dishon, S.; Miller, A. Internet usage by patients with multiple sclerosis: Implications to participatory medicine and personalized healthcare. *Mult. Scler. Int.* **2010**, *2010*, 640749. [CrossRef]
25. Feigin, V.L.; Vos, T.; Nichols, E.; Owolabi, M.O.; Carroll, W.M.; Dichgans, M.; Deuschl, G.; Parmar, P.; Brainin, M.; Murray, C. The global burden of neurological disorders: Translating evidence into policy. *Lancet Neurol.* **2020**, *19*, 255–265. [CrossRef]
26. Dorsey, E.R.; Constantinescu, R.; Thompson, J.P.; Biglan, K.M.; Holloway, R.G.; Kieburtz, K.; Marshall, F.J.; Ravina, B.M.; Schifitto, G.; Siderowf, A.; et al. Projected number of people with Parkinson disease in the most populous nations, 2005 through 2030. *Neurology* **2007**, *68*, 384–386. [CrossRef]
27. Walton, C.; King, R.; Rechtman, L.; Kaye, W.; Leray, E.; Marrie, R.A.; Robertson, N.; la Rocca, N.; Uitdehaag, B.; van der Mei, I.; et al. Rising prevalence of multiple sclerosis worldwide: Insights from the Atlas of MS, third edition. *Mult. Scler.* **2020**, *26*, 1816–1821. [CrossRef] [PubMed]
28. Marrie, R.A.; Elliott, L.; Marriott, J.; Cossoy, M.; Blanchard, J.; Leung, S.; Yu, N. Effect of comorbidity on mortality in multiple sclerosis. *Neurology* **2015**, *85*, 240–247. [CrossRef]
29. Moccia, M.; Lanzillo, R.; Brescia Morra, V.; Bonavita, S.; Tedeschi, G.; Leocani, L.; Lavorgna, L. Assessing disability and relapses in multiple sclerosis on tele-neurology. *Neurol. Sci.* **2020**, *41*, 1369–1371. [CrossRef]
30. Bevan, C.; Crabtree, E.; Zhao, C.; Gomez, R.; Garcha, P.; Morrissey, J.; Dierkhising, J.; Green, A.J.; Hauser, S.L.; AC Cree, B.; et al. Toward a low-cost, in-home, telemedicine-enabled assessment of disability in multiple sclerosis. *Mult. Scler.* **2019**, *25*, 1526–1534.
31. Atreja, A.; Mehta, N.; Miller, D.; Moore, S.; Nichols, K.; Miller, H.; Harris, C.M. One size does not fit all: Using qualitative methods to inform the development of an Internet portal for multiple sclerosis patients. *AMIA Annu. Symp. Proc.* **2005**, *2005*, 16–20.
32. Settle, J.R.; Maloni, H.W.; Bedra, M.; Finkelstein, J.; Zhan, M.; Wallin, M.T. Monitoring medication adherence in multiple sclerosis using a novel web-based tool: A pilot study. *J. Telemed. Telecare* **2016**, *22*, 225–233. [CrossRef] [PubMed]
33. Strowd, R.E.; Strauss, L.; Graham, R.; Dodenhoff, K.; Schreiber, A.; Thomson, S.; Ambrosini, A.; Thurman, A.M.; Olszewski, C.; Smith, L.D.; et al. Rapid implementation of outpatient teleneurology in rural Appalachia: Barriers and disparities. *Neurol. Clin. Pract.* **2020**, *11*, 232–241. [CrossRef] [PubMed]
34. Cummings, C.; Almallouhi, E.; Al Kasab, S.; Spiotta, A.M.; Holmstedt, C.A. Brief report: Blacks are less likely to present with strokes during the COVID-19 pandemic: Observations from the buckle of the stroke belt. *Stroke* **2020**, *51*, 3107–3111. [CrossRef] [PubMed]
35. Plow, M.; Motl, R.W.; Finlayson, M.; Bethoux, F. Response heterogeneity in a randomized controlled trial of telerehabilitation interventions among adults with multiple sclerosis. *J. Telemed. Telecare* **2020**. [CrossRef] [PubMed]

MDPI
St. Alban-Anlage 66
4052 Basel
Switzerland
Tel. +41 61 683 77 34
Fax +41 61 302 89 18
www.mdpi.com

Journal of Personalized Medicine Editorial Office
E-mail: jpm@mdpi.com
www.mdpi.com/journal/jpm

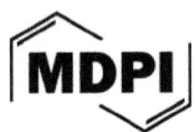

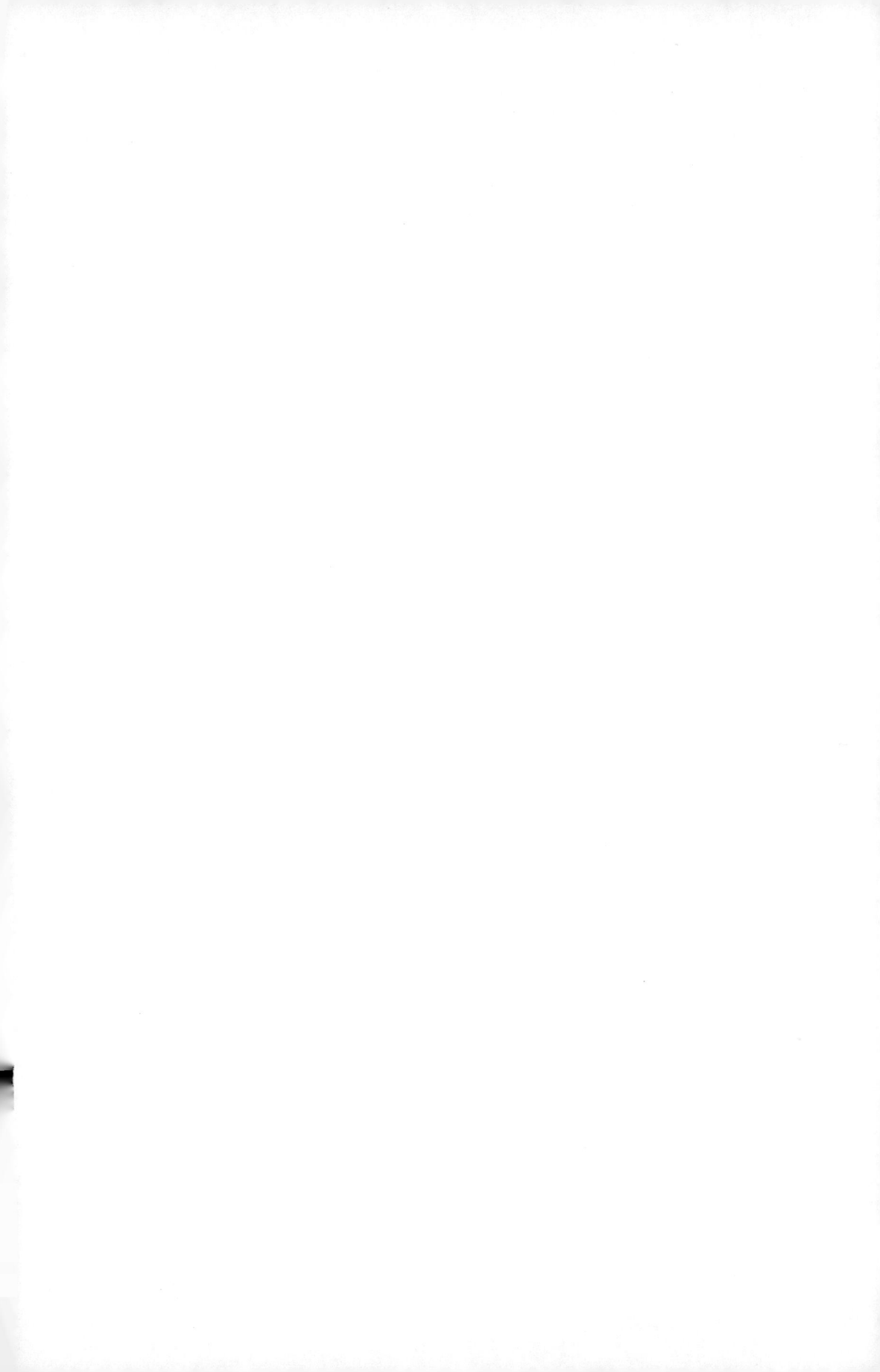

www.ingramcontent.com/pod-product-compliance
Lightning Source LLC
LaVergne TN
LVHW070553100526
838202LV00012B/451